Preface:

If you are reading this then you might be looking to make a change in your life. This could be to lose weight, to get in better shape, to improve your quality of life or learn a little about health and nutrition. Starting this journey can seem like a daunting task, and you might not know where to begin. Something I have noticed over the years is that when reading about diets and exercises topics the authors tend to operate on the assumption that you already know what they are talking about. You will run into words and concepts that you don't fully understand. This can lead you to misunderstanding what the author is trying to convey to you and cause you to apply the information incorrectly, or feel lost. Before you know it you are frustrated because you think you are doing everything correctly and it's just not working, when in reality the author just did a poor job of making the information understandable to the average person who doesn't have advanced degrees in health and fitness.

That's where this book comes in. Within these pages you will find information on health topics, nutrition, facts and myths related to wellness/fitness, and tips and tricks to live a healthier life. This book is designed to take these complex topics and break them down into brief easily understandable sections. There are 182 topics covered and the design is for one topic to be read every day, and over the course of the next 6 month you will create a healthier life style with one small step a day. Think of it as a daily devotional to a healthier you. Some of the topics covered might already be known to you, while some provide new information. The goal of this book is for you to gain and apply the knowledge over a longer period of time. Allowing you to make small easily sustainable changes over the months, this will allow you to ease into the changes and keep building on them one day at a time. Making small changes overtime will help you to stick with them, unlike the rapid sudden changes used in crash dieting.

As you read through this book you will more than likely become aware of a simple fact. I am not a writer, I am a health teacher. You might (will) find a variety of grammatical errors in this book, all I ask is that you look past my short comings as a writer and focus on what you can learn. So welcome to the first step to achieving a healthier you.

1.

Calories

We are going to start out this book with a topic that will lay the ground work for a healthy life style. We are going to take a look at what exactly a calorie is and what your body does with it. Simply put a calorie is a unit of measurement for energy contained in the food we eat. They are not something that we can just physically remove, and we can't just avoid them all together because we need them to power our bodies. Think of it like putting gas in your car, without the gas your car wouldn't run and much like the car our bodies cannot run without calories.

Where does the energy in a calorie come from? The myth is that calories are a separate thing from the other well known nutrients such as fat and protein. The truth is that a calorie is actually a combination of the nutrients found in all of the foods we eat. Calories are locked in the fats, proteins, and carbohydrates of the foods we consume. Think of it as a blanket term that accounts for all of the energy stored in food. As your body digests these nutrients the energy from them is released and used to fuel our metabolisms. A metabolism is simply defined as "The chemical processes that occur within a living organism in order to maintain life."

So now we know that a calorie is simply a unit of energy used to fuel our bodies and it is made up of a combination of the nutrients found in our foods. Now how does this relate to the body system and weight loss/gain? Looking back at the car analogy from earlier you can only fit so much gas in a car before it becomes full and no more can be added to it until some of the gas is used to run the engine. Unfortunately your body does not operate the same. When we have consumed enough calories to run our bodies there is no real function to tell us that we have had enough. Instead our bodies will store the extra calories consumed, in our fat tissues to be used later if our bodies are in need of energy and not enough calories are consumed to meet our metabolic needs. If you eat more calories than your body needs you will gain weight in the form of fat, if you do not consume enough calories then your body will rely on the energy in your fat stores to run your body. A calorie in vs a calorie out is what it all boils down to.

A calorie is a calorie is a calorie, your body does not burn a calorie from a steak any different than a calorie from a hot-fudge Sunday. This is a very important point and something that should be guiding your journey and the reason I put it at the start of the book. Remember a calorie is a combination of all the nutrients in your food so it is always the same when used by your body. Think of it this way, your TV uses power from an energy source, for most of us that energy source is the electric company. That electric company probably uses a variety of methods to create that energy. It could be a coal powered plant, solar powered, or a wind turbine. No matter what the method for generating the energy is, the end product is all the same and your TV cannot tell the difference from what source the energy comes from. Your body is the same; a calorie is a unit of energy no matter where it comes from. That's not to say there isn't a big difference in the types of nutrients that make up the calories and those nutrients effects on the body. However that is a subject to be covered on another day.

To start out this journey on the right foot your task for this section is to start looking at the total amount of calories you are consuming for each meal over the next several days. I am not asking you to change your dietary choices at this time, eat as you normally would. Just pay close attention to how many calories you are eating, remember to look at portion sizes (we will cover this in detail later), and write it down. The total might surprise you.

2.

Metabolism Explained

I am sure we have all heard the term metabolism but what does it really mean? I mentioned it in the Calories section; the definition is "The chemical processes that occur within a living organism in order to maintain life." So broken down it is the process of converting calories consumed to energy to be used or stored. Your metabolism will also draw on fat reserves when the body is operating in a calorie deficit. For this section metabolism is as simple as the burning of calories and the rate at which they are burnt.

Have you ever heard the excuse "I have a slow metabolism" or "you're so lucky that you have a fast metabolism."? Be honest, have you yourself ever used this excuse? What if I was to tell you that technically speaking the bigger you are the faster your metabolism actually is. The truth is that it takes more calories to sustain an overweight person than it does to sustain a person of normal weight. Let's dive a little deeper into this idea.

We all have a BMR, this is the Basal Metabolic Rate. Basically your BMR is the amount of calories you need to run your body systems and that's it, movement and activity level is not taken into account. Your BMR can be estimated using the Harris-Benedict equation. There are many options available to us in the modern age where we can hop on our cell phones or computers and plug some numbers into it and get our BMR but we are going to go over how to figure it out ourselves. This is important because the methods used in apps or websites could be different, or give you inaccurate results. This formula was first published in 1918, but we will be using the updated form which is as follows:

Men: BMR = 66 + (6.23 X weight in pounds) + (12.7 X height in inches) – (6.8 X age)

Women: BMR = 655 + (4.35 X weight in pounds) + (4.7 X height in inches) – (4.7 X age)

I am going to quickly cover two different examples and for the sake of reading time the two examples will just be male; however the same principle will apply to both genders. So let's assume that we have two males of equal height of 6ft tall and equal age of 30 years old. Male 1 weighs 165 pounds, while male 2 weighs 285 pounds. Running those numbers through the BMR formula we get male 1 with a BMR of 1,804 calories, and male 2 with a BMR of 2,551 calories. This means in a 24 hour period male 1 would burn 1,804 calories just to run his body systems, while male 2 will burn 2,551 calories just to run his body systems in the same time period. That is a difference of 747 calories, which means that in order for male 2 to burn 747 more calories in a 24 hour period his metabolism would have to be running at a "faster" rate than his smaller counterpart. So as you can see the slower metabolism being the reason for weight gain is a myth.

Remember your BMR is just the base amount of calories you need, and your total calories burnt will be higher due to the energy we use when we go for a walk or workout. Any physical activity we do consumes calories, some activities like jumping rope burn a lot of calories while others like walking or standing burn fewer calories. So how do you figure out how many calories you actually burn throughout the day? It's pretty easy actually but you will need to figure out your BMR first. Ok so now you have your BMR we are going to find out your Total Daily Energy Expenditure (TDEE). TDEE can be broken down into 5 categories based on how much physical activity you engage in in a day. Those categories are Sedentary, Lightly Active, Moderately Active, Very Active and Extremely Active. Broken down those categories can be classified as follows:

Sedentary: Little to no exercise, desk job, most of the day spent sitting or not moving much

- TDEE = 1.2xBMR

Lightly Active: Very light exercise, make a small effort to not be sitting all day.

- TDEE = 1.375xBMR

Moderately active: You make an effort to be active, might hit the gym a little or go for walks often

- TDEE= 1.55xBMR

Very Active: You exercise heavily everyday, you might have a very physical job, you make your fitness a priority in your life.

- TDEE = 1.725xBMR

Extremely active: Very heavy exercise routine/physical job. Likely an athlete or you exercise several times a day.

- TDEE = 1.9xBMR

The truth is that anyone reading this book likely falls into one of the first 3 categories. Now we will use these categories to determine TDEE. You will select which category you fall into then use the multiplying factor with your BMR to find out your estimated Total Daily Energy Expenditure. So if you are lightly active you will use the numbers above, take your BMR and multiply it by the lightly active multiplying factor of 1.375. This will give you your estimated calories burnt per day counting exercise.

Let's return to our two male examples from earlier. For this example we will say that male 1 falls into the Moderately Active category, while male 2 falls into the sedentary category. So returning to their BMR's we calculated earlier let's find their TDEE's.

Male 1: BMR is 1,804 now multiply by the activity factor for moderately active which is 1.55 and you get: TDEE = 1,804x1.55 = 2,796 calories.

Male 2: BMR is 2,551 now multiply by the activity factor for sedentary which is 1.2 and you get: TDEE = 2,551x1.2 = 3,061 calories.

As you can see male 1 increased the number of calories burned during the day by just shy of 1,000 calories, while male 2 burned an extra 510 calories through activity. If male 2 were to increase their activity to the same level as male 1 their total calories burnt during the day would be 3,954 calories. That is an increase of nearly 1,000 calories burnt!

To finish up this section, metabolism is simply the energy our bodies' burn, and that energy comes in the form of calories. It is possible to increase your calories burnt and therefor increase your metabolism through activity, and you are able to estimate your BMR and TDEE through the formulas we went over above. Knowing how many calories you burn in a single day helps you to be able to plan how many calories you need to consume to lose weight, gain weight, or remain at your current weight. Eating fewer calories than your TDEE will result in weight loss while eating more than your TDEE will result in weight gain. Now that you are already starting to monitor how many calories you are consuming in a given day you will be able to compare those total calories to your TDEE and see if you are eating properly to gain/lose weight. It is important to be honest with yourself about your activity level! If you over estimate you will be reducing your ability to get an accurate reading on how many calories you need in a day. This can greatly affect your success going forward.

3.

What is Fat?

Welcome back, so far we have taken a look at two subjects that relate to body fat. It is time for us to dive into what fat actually is in the body. You may hear fat being referred to as adipose tissue as well. The simple definition of adipose tissue is a kind of body tissue containing stored fat that serves as a source of energy. For this section though we will be referring to body fat candidly as fat.

We already know that fat is produced in the body when you consume more calories than your body burns for that day. Over time if you regularly consume more calories than you need a large amount of body fat is produced. Just how many calories do you need to overeat by to produce a single pound of fat? Well, there are a total of 3,500 calories in a single pound of fat. That seems like it is a lot of calories! The truth is it is not a lot of calories when you think about it. Let's look at it over a period of a year, if you were to over eat on average by just 100 calories a day (That's a single medium banana for perspective) after a year you would have overeaten by 36,500 calories. Let's break that down then by dividing it by the total calories in a pound of fat, which is 3,500 calories. You get just over 10 pounds of fat accumulated on your body in a single year. So next let's spread that out over a 5 year span, that's 10 pounds of fat gained every year for 5 years. You are looking at 50 pounds of fat gained, just by simply over eating by an average of 100 calories a day!

So if your reading this book because you have put on some weight over the years and you are looking at a way to get rid of those unwanted pounds, it is time to be honest with yourself. Did you slowly gain weight over a series of years; you didn't just wake up 50 pounds heavier one morning? When you first started putting on weight did you start to notice it as a slow steady gain of 10-20 pounds a year? Chances are that you, like most people did a slow steady gain of weight over the period of several years. This is often due to as we get older we don't "play" and be as active as we did when we were younger, we become more sedentary with our jobs and our home life. So our activity level drops but the amount of food we eat stays steady or increases. So what you use to eat as a kid was burned off by your more active life style while your more sedentary life style results in those calories being stored as fat.

Have you ever heard the phrase "a pound of muscle weighs more than a pound of fat"? I have always found this phrase annoying, but I understand the idea behind it. Although a pound of fat and a pound of muscle weigh the same on a scale, they look drastically different when compared in size. A pound of fat is about the size of a standard can of vegetables, or about the size of a large fist. A single pound of muscle is about half that size. So a pound of muscle doesn't weight more than a pound of fat it is just more dense and takes up less area.

There are a few different types of fat within the body and some serve purposes beyond energy storage, while others can lead to unhealthy bodies and disease. The two main types we will be discussing are visceral fat, and subcutaneous fat.

Visceral fat is commonly referred to as abdominal fat because it can be found in the abdominal cavity. The abdominal cavity is the hollow within your body where all of your organs are housed. As you can imagine there is not a great deal of space left in your abdominal cavity after when you account for the space occupied by your organs like the heart, lungs, stomach, and intestines. Visceral fat fills up the space left between the organs and can even surround organs such as the heart. If you think that sounds bad well you would be correct. Having a high amount of visceral fat can lead to several health concerns such as increased likelihood of heart attack, certain cancers and type 2 diabetes. A specific type of visceral fat to be wary of is Epicedial fat, also known as the fat that specifically surrounds your heart. Having too much of this type could disrupt the functions of your heart, like beating.

The visceral fat is more common in men due to a difference in sex hormones between the two genders. It can often cause the "belly fat" which is when the abdomen protrudes excessively; this is often referred to as the beer gut. Now for women you are more disposed to store your body fat in the hips, legs, and buttocks. However as you age and your estrogen hormones begin to decrease the fat begins to "migrate" towards your abdomen, causing you to develop the protruding abdomen and risk of medical issues. Keep in mind that everyone has some visceral fat in their abdominal cavity because it can serve a purpose like being a protective cushion for organs, but excessive cushion could cause harm to those same organs.

The other type of fat that is important to mention is subcutaneous fat. This is the fat that is located under the skin but above the muscle tissue. This is the fat that you are able to more or less see on a person. This could cause you to have a chubby face or arms, it is what causes the "spare tires" around our mid regions and causes our clothes to no longer fit as we gain more and more weight. The health concerns as a result of this type of fat are not a dire as the visceral fat, but that doesn't mean there are not risks to your health, or your mental health and self-body image.

So at this point you have begun to monitor your calories consumed each day and have even found your TDEE. Now I want you to start thinking about it in terms of time. Are you finding that you have been consuming more calories than you burn in a day? Do you think you have been consuming more calories than you need on average over several years? Look back on your experience over the last several years; does the weight gain seem to follow a trend of over eating by a little? Over a long period of time a small amount of over eating extended over a long period of time can add up to a lot of weight gain.

4.

Portion Control

Moving right along now it is time to tackle a subject that can be difficult to solve, portion control. Portion control can be a difficult thing to fully understand because portion size can change drastically between the various foods we consume. Being able to read and apply portion sizes to the foods we eat will be key to both short and long term weight loss as well as weight control. We are also going to take a look at a few items that can be used to aid you along this journey.

First lets define what portion control is. For the sake of this book it can be defined as "a method of monitoring food intake to fall within the prescribed calorie content of the food or diet". The food that we buy typically comes with a nutritional label, and on that label you will find a breakdown of everything that is in that food. The total carbs, proteins, sugars, vitamins and so on. For this section we are only going to focus on the calorie count and the recommended portion size, we will cover the whole nutritional label in a later section. So let's look at an example:

Nutrition Facts

Serving Size 3 oz. (85g)
Serving Per Container 2

Amount Per Serving

Calories 200	Calories from Fat 120

	% Daily Value*
Total Fat 15g	**20 %**
Saturated Fat 5g	**28 %**
Trans Fat 3g	
Cholesterol 30mg	**10 %**
Sodium 650mg	**28 %**
Total Carbohydrate 30g	**10 %**
Dietary Fiber 0g	**0 %**
Sugars 5g	
Protein 5g	

Vitamin A 5%	•	Vitamin C 2%
Calcium 15%	•	Iron 5%

*Percent Daily Values are based on a 2,000 calorie diet. Your Daily Values may be higher or lower depending on your calorie needs.

	Calories	2,000	2,500
Total Fat	Less than	65g	80g
Sat Fat	Less than	20g	25g
Cholesterol	Less than	300mg	300mg
Sodium	Less than	2,400mg	2,400mg
Total Carbohydrate		300mg	375mg
Dietary Fiber		25g	30g

Looking at the nutritional label above we can see all of the information about the food. We are going to focus on the "Serving Size", "Serving Per Container", and "Calories". Which are the first 3 options. Up first the serving size, which here is 3 oz. That can be a difficult thing to estimate by looking at it or without a food scale. However there are some context clues on the label that can help you to estimate the amount that is a serving. Here we can go to the "Servings Per Container" section of the label. This will tell you the total servings that are in whatever the container might be such as a can or a box. For this the servings per container is 2. So using that information we can now get a good estimate on how much a single serving will be. If there are 2 servings in the container then a single serving is half of all of the food. Easy enough, this technique can be applied if the serving per container is different. For example, if the serving per container is 3 then you would know that a single serving is 1/3 of the total volume of food. Back to this label, since we know that a single serving is half of the total amount of food next we need to find out how many calories are in a single serving. Looking at the label you need to find the "Calories" line and trace it over to find the number of calories. For this label it is 200 calories per serving. Now we know that if you eat half of the total amount of food in this example you will have consumed 1 portion and 200 calories.

Continuing with this example you can see that it is really easy to over eat and think you only consumed 200 calories when you really could have consumed up to 400 if you ate the whole container. Let's put this in perspective, let's pretend that the food this label represents is a type of fish. 3oz of fish is roughly the size of a deck of playing cards. When was the last time you ate a piece of fish that small? Think back to the "what is fat" section we covered earlier this week.

Remember how a little bit of over eating by only a few hundred calories or less a day can add up to 10's of pounds in a single year. This is where portion control becomes such a great skill to develop, knowing your portion sizes allows you to accurately monitor your calorie intake. When you can accurately account for the total calories that you are consuming then you will have a better understanding of how much you can eat and remain in a calorie deficit if you are trying to lose weight.

It all comes down to math; I once heard a saying that goes something like this. If someone tells you that they only eat 500 calories a day and they still gain weight, and someone else says they eat 5000 calories a day and never gain a single pound, then I can show you two people who are bad at math. This meaning that they don't know how to properly count their calories. Typically people are found to overestimate portion size and under estimate calorie content. This will always lead to frustration and giving up on their weight loss goal, because in their mind they are doing it right and not overeating. However what they are really doing is shooting themselves in the foot by not taking portion control seriously.

Don't believe me? Let's take a look at a study done by *Sue D. Pedersen, MD, FRCPC; Jian Kang, MSc; Gregory A. Kline, MD, FRCPC.* They conducted a study titled *"Portion Control Plate for Weight Loss in Obese Patients With Type 2 Diabetes Mellitus. A Controlled Clinical Trial"* Now as you can see they tested subjects with diabetes; the results would be the same with or without diabetes. The study used a control group who tried to lose weight on their own and a test group who used special commercially available portion control plates to control their food intake. A portion control plate is a special plate that is sectioned off to provide the correct portion size for foods like meat, vegetables, bread/carbs and so on. So the idea is that you place the food you are eating into the portion slot and if it fills it up then the portion is correct, if it goes over then the portion is too big.

The study found that the group that used the portion control plates lost a significant larger amount of weight in 6 months than the control group. They also had the added benefit of seeing a reduction in the need of their medications. This forced portion control allowed them to select the correct amount of food to meet their daily calorie goals and lose more weight than those who were left to figure out portion control on their own.

All that being said you do not need special plates to understand portion control, but the study shows that it can make it easier, now we are going to take a look at a few options out their along with a portion control guide. Up first we have the portion control plates that were mentioned in the study. There are a variety of options for this and you can get them in all sorts of styles to match your food choices. There is also the option that is similar to the portion plates, this is the portion control cups. These special cups can be used like a standard measuring cup but instead of measuring a ½ cup or ¾ cup like a standard measuring cup, they are specific to a type of food. So you might have a cup for pastas or vegetables, where you simply fill the specific cup that matches the food and get a correct portion. Then you just dump the food out on a standard plate and now you have the correct portion.

The final trick I am going to talk about when discussing portion control is rough size estimations, and here are a few examples. A cup of broccoli is about the size of a baseball, while a ½ cup of fruit is the size of a tennis ball. Half of a small bagel is the size of a hockey puck while a ½ cup serving of of pasta is also about the size of a hockey puck. Finally a teaspoon of something like butter is about the size of a single die. I added this part not to give you a comprehensive list of food comparisons but to show you that you can develop these methods for yourself. Look at what you eat and make your own portion size comparisons.

There will be times that you are out and eating at let's say a party, and you are deciding on how much of a certain food to put on your plate. If you have something to compare a serving size to in your head then you can get a rough estimate on the serving size you have and the calorie count. So as you begin to focus on your portions and serving sizes take a mental note of how big that serving is and maybe compare it to something for future reference. It might just keep you from over eating in the future.

Now that we know about portion sizes and their importance to your calorie intake it is time to apply it. So at this time you have already started to monitor your calorie intake for each day. Now I want you to really focus on your portion sizes when counting calories. You might be surprised to find out that you might have been way off on the amount of calories you thought you were consuming and the actual amount you were eating. All because you were incorrect on your portion estimations.

5

Truth about Diet

We have been going at a steady pace going over nutritional information but have not covered much in the way of diets and exercise. There is a reason for this, building a base knowledge is important to having a full understanding of how to achieve and maintain a healthy body and life style. Here we are going to talk about diets in this section and what you need to know about the term diet.

The term diet can be used to mean two very different things; in fact you might not have been sure of which meaning I was using in the first paragraph. The first definition is "the kinds of food that a person, animal, or community habitually eats". The second definition is "a special course of food to which one restricts oneself, either to lose weight or for medical reasons." As you can see the term diet can mean just what food you eat or it can have the definition of being a means of restricting certain foods, this definition lends itself to be a temporary behavior. I prefer to use the first definition as it is more accurate for the information that I cover, when I am referring to the action of restricting food choices in the form of a "diet" I will refer to it as "restrictive diet". Now that we understand the terms let's move forward.

Take a moment and think of all of the restrictive diets that you have heard about or have actively participated in. Some of the big ones could be the Atkins diet, the grape fruit diet, low carb diet, and so on. What do all of these diets have in common? Simple, they restrict you from eating certain foods or to only eating certain foods for a short period of time. Restrictive dieting is a temporary function that is used to reach a goal. The truth is that weight loss can and usually does occur when you enter into one of these restrictive diets. The problem though is that the restrictive diet is again a temporary change in your dietary behavior. Let's say that you give a low carb diet a go, so you are restricting the amount of carbohydrates that you are consuming. Carbohydrates if you recall are one of the components of a calorie, but do you know what a carbohydrate (carb for short) is? A carb is the combination of the sugars, starches and dietary fibers found in our foods. You can have complex carbs and simple carbs, but we will deal with that in a later section. A carbohydrate contains the various versions of sugars in our foods, and as we know our bodies rely on a balance of sugar to keep us running, think blood sugar levels.

Having your blood sugar levels get to low can cause you to become tired, irritable, and lethargic. While having blood sugar levels to high can cause harm to your organs, and cause you to be jittery followed by an eventual sugar high crash, where your blood sugar drops. So as you can see you need to eat carbs, but you need to have a balance. Having a healthy balance of foods and nutrients in your daily diets allows you to maintain the nutritional needs of your body to operate at its best. When you restrict or remove nutrients that the body needs then you can disrupt its normal functions.

This is why I am covering the restrictive diets now, you have already learned about calories, fat, metabolism, and portion control. Understanding that you can lose weight without a restrictive diet where any one food or food group is removed is essential to moving forward and having long term success. If you practice proper portion size and remain in your calorie range you will lose weight, and you can do it without cutting out entire food groups. This practice is often referred to as a "life style change".

When you commit to a life style change, in this context, you are actively changing behaviors that you engage in for your life span. This is where restrictive diets and life style changes differ. In a restrictive diet you will eventually get tired of only eating certain foods or not being allowed to eat the foods you love. Once you become tired of the restrictions you have placed on yourself then you have a high probability or resorting back to your old dietary habits. I am sure that you have heard the idea that that diets always fail and most people gain all the weight back within 5 years. Well that is for the most part true! However looking at what we have already learned what could be the cause of this? Take a moment and really apply what we have learned already, this is an important step. Simply reading my words won't get you to your goal, you need to be able to apply the information too. The reason why people gain the weight back after the restrictive diet is because they complete the diet either through becoming tired of it or reaching their goal. Once they stop restricting what they eat and return back to normal eating habits then the trend of slowly overeating begins to happen again. Once you return to the same old habits that put you in the position that made you want to start a restrictive diet, you will begin gaining the weight back slowly overtime. Remember in the fat section how just averaging over eating by 100 calories a day over a period of 5 years can add up to 50 or more pounds. This is where the "all diets fail" idea comes into a reality.

In a life style change you are changing those over eating behaviors not by restricting the types of foods you eat but by reducing the overall calories that you consume. This allows you to continue to eat the foods you like, as long as you are accounting for how many calories you should be eating in a day. This promotes a lasting change and will help you to maintain at a goal weight for years to come. As a result, this is why I always advocate for a life style change and educating yourself about health and nutrition. Restrictive diets might serve a purpose for a short term weight loss goal, but overall you will be putting stress on yourself both physically and mentally for something that has a high failure rate.

There is a consequence though to the life style change of counting calories and portion control. You will eventually begin to gravitate to healthy food options! This is because of the volume differences that you will begin to see in portions of equal calories. For perspective on this, according to the McDonalds nutritional chart a quarter pounder with cheese contains 530 calories. That does not include a drink or sides, just the sandwich itself. For the sake of this example assume your calorie goal for the day is 1800 calories; let's add up all of the calories from a standard MacDonald's meal. For a medium meal of a drink, the burger and the fries you are looking at 1,080 calories. This means that you would only have a total of 720 calories left in your plan for the day. Now you can always budget and allow for the calories to be used on eating here and there, but in the long run it can become very difficult to stave off hunger if you're eating high calorie fast food regularly then reducing other meals substantially to stay within your daily calorie range. Choosing foods that are of the more "healthy" variety can allow you to eat a greater volume while keeping calorie count low. Below is a list of just some random healthy food choices I selected and their calorie count.

Bagged Salad 1.5 cups	15 calories
Steak 6 ounces	460 calories
Egg	78 calories
Banana	106 calories
Baby Spinach leaves ½ cup	7 calories
Carrots 1 cup	45 calories
Cooked Brown Rice 1 cup	216 calories
Quinoa ½ cup	111 calories

Adding all of those foods up you will see that combined they equal 1,038 calories while also providing a large variety of nutrients and vitamins. Take note of the total volume of food as well, that is far more food volume than the single McDonald's meal presented above. Eating the healthier options and taking note of the correct portions and calorie content can allow you to eat more filling meals whereas blowing you calorie budget on high calorie options can lead to lower food volume and the return of the hunger feeling quickly.

You should now be beginning to understand that nutritional choices you make are important, and for any long term success you will need to understand portion sizes and calorie count. You do not need to starve yourself to lose weight, as I shown you above you can eat a very filling amount of food as long as you are selecting the proper foods. You can also step off the healthy food train occasionally but you need to be sure you are accounting for the total calories consumed and adjusting accordingly to stay within your daily calorie range. The choice is up to you, you can continue to use restrictive diets and see weight loss followed by weight gain. Or you can decide today to commit to what you have learned so far about life style changes and how to properly account for your calorie choices. I will begin to introduce exercise concepts occasionally in the following sections, but remember you can never outrun a bad diet.

6
Target Heart Rate

We have spent the first week learning about how to understand what caused weight gain and the best way to reverse it from a dietary stand point. Controlling your diets is the biggest step you will need to take on this journey, and it's going to be difficult but with commitment you will see progress and it will become easier. We are now going to begin let's call it phase 2, which is to understand the importance of engaging in regular physical activity. The first step to this is to understand your target heart rate.

Starting with the basics, your heart is a muscle and like any other muscle it can become stronger when it is exercised or worked out. As your heart becomes stronger your beats per minute (bpm) begins to drop, this is due to the heart being able to pump more blood out to the systems of your body per contraction. Essentially working out your heart allows it to be more efficient per contraction or pump. But why does the heart pump, and why does it have to increase its bpm during activity? Our muscles and organs need oxygen to function, and as these systems consume oxygen they create waste in the form of carbon dioxide. Blood is pumped through the heart that carries both the needed oxygen and the waste products. The heart has 4 chambers to it, the right atrium, the right ventricle, the left atrium, and the left ventricle. Let's start with the right atrium, blood without oxygen (deoxygenated blood) containing the waste product carbon dioxide enters into the right atrium. From there it is moved into the right ventricle, and when the heart contracts (pumps) that blood is sent to the lungs through the pulmonary artery. In the lungs the blood releases the carbon dioxide and loads up on the oxygen becoming oxygenated. We then exhale the carbon dioxide through our normal breathing.

From the lungs the blood is sent through the pulmonary vein to the left atrium, and then moved to the left ventricle. From here the oxygen rich blood is pumped out through the aorta to all the systems of your body. This includes your organs, muscles, brain, and skin and so on. The process then repeats, as your organs remove the oxygen from your blood they replace it with the waste product and send it back to the heart in the vena cava which leads back to the right atrium.

Your body responds to physical activity by increasing the rate at which your heart pumps blood. It does this because as you exercise your muscles increase their workload and need to consume more oxygen to function properly. As a result they increase their carbon dioxide production as well, carbon dioxide is toxic to the body so it needs to be released and exhaled out of the lungs. This is why your heart rate will speed up and your breathing becomes faster and deeper to meet the demands of the body. This process is known as your cardiorespiratory system.

Now let's talk about your target heart rate and what that actually means. Like your other muscles there is a point where the exercise is benefiting you and there is a point where it really is not. For example if you were doing bicep curls but you were only curling a 1 pound weight 3 times a day, you would likely see no benefits or improvements from it. If you were curling 15 pounds a day for 3 sets of 15 repetitions then you would likely see improvements to your muscle strength. Your heart works in the same way, if you work it out to easy then it will have no reason to improve itself. Both skeletal muscles and cardiac (heart) muscles grow and become stronger when you apply stress to them, the stress can be in the form of an exercise. Over time your body will increase the strength of the muscles to respond to that stress (exercise), so that it becomes easier on you.

When you work out your heart you should try to keep your heart rate in a certain range of beats per minute for a specific time frame. The range is known as your target heart rate zone. How do you figure out what your target heart rate is? Well it is actually pretty simple, but it will take some prep. First we need to find your resting heart rate, this is the beats per minute that your heart does when you are completely relaxed and resting. The best time to check for your resting heart rate is first thing in the morning before you even get out of bed. What you do is take your pointer and middle fingers and find your pulse, you can use either your radial artery located on your wrist just below the thumb. Or you can find it on your carotid artery which is located on either side of your throat. Once you find your pulse you will count how many beats you feel for a specific time frame. What I like to do is count the beats I feel for 30 seconds then just multiply the number I get by 2. This will give you how many beats per minute during rest, also known as your resting heart rate. For example if I felt 31 beats in 30 seconds then I would take 31 X 2 = 61 bpm.

The next parts for finding your target heart rate is a little more complicated, but still easy. We now need to find your maximum heart rate; this is the highest you should ever let your heart rate get. To find this you simply take 220 – your age. So for me I take 220 – 29yrs old = 191 bpm. So my max heart rate is 191 beat per minute, take a moment and find yours. Next take your max heart rate and subtract your resting heart rate from it. Save that number it is called your Heart Rate Reserve

(HRR). Now take your HRR number and multiply it by .6, this will give you 60% of your HRR. Next take your original HRR number again and multiply it by .85, this will give you 85% of your HRR. Now we take the 60% HRR number and add your original resting heart rate number to it, then do the same with the 85% HRR number. This will give you a low end of 60 percent of your target heart rate and a high end of 85% of your target heart zone.

For me it looks like this:

- Resting heart rate = 60 bpm
- Max heart rate is 220 − 29 = 191 bpm
- HRR is 191 − 60 (resting heart rate) = 131 HRR
- 131 X .6 = 79 (60% of my HRR)
- 131 X .85 = 105 (85% of my HRR)
- 79 + 60 (resting heart rate) = 139 (60 % of max heart rate)
- 105 + 60 (resting heart rate) = 165 (85% of max heart rate)

So my target heart rate range is between 139 beat per minute and 165 beat per minute. This is considered the optimal range I should exercise my heart at to get the best results, and improve my heart strength as well as burn calories. So when deciding to engage in physical activity you can try to get into that range to really improve your heart health and get the most out of your exercise. However this is a slow process, you need to ease into any exercise program, it is ok and recommended that you start slow and build up to your target heart rate. You might not be able to get yourself into that range, yet. Over time though, you will see that you are improving and moving towards being able to exercise in that range. You will come to learn and apply the power of "yet". I can't do something….. Yet. Yet tells you that might not be able to do something at this time, but that you are working towards achieving your goals.

Now that you know your target heart rate and understand the importance of it, we need to know how long to stay in the target heart rate zone. It is recommended that you exercise in that zone for 20 to 30 minutes. I know that seems like a huge mountain to climb, but if you start out small and slowly work your way up to it you will be there before you know it. Right now you might only be able to walk a short distance, that's ok. Walk that short distance, then increase that distance a little and a little more then a little more. Soon that distance is not short at all anymore. Then you can increase the pace, and remember what we just learned about increasing the stress on your body? Your heart will increase to meet the demand. Soon you will be in your target heart rate zone!

There are thing out there that can aide you in tracking your heart rate during exercise. Wearable devices such as smart watches and Fitbit are everywhere. I am not sponsored by any of these products, however I do own a Fitbit that I use to track my heart rate and I have found it to be a big help. Although I enjoy using my wearable device it is by no means needed, tracking your heart rate can be done in a minute just by counting your pulse. Wearable devices that do it for you are a luxury not a necessity, if you chose to use one that is up to you. We will cover them in detail in a later section! So for now use what you learned to discover your target heart rate zone, it will come in handy during this journey we are taking together!

The 5 components of Fitness

Becoming a healthier fit person can be difficult, and there is a misconception that working out or exercising has to be running on a treadmill for hours or becoming a gym bro and lifting things up and putting them back down. The truth is that you don't have to be a treadmill bunny or a gym bro to be fit. Finding a physical activity that fits your interests and abilities is important, and will help to keep you motivated to continue participating in them. In this section we will be covering the 5 components to fitness and a brief over view of what each of them means. They are cardiorespiratory endurance, muscular strength, muscular endurance, flexibility, and body composition.

Cardiorespiratory endurance was hinted at in the prior target heart rate section, so we already know a little about it. We know that Cardiorespiratory is the function of your heart and lungs working to supply the systems of the body with the oxygen and energy that they need to function at their best. Within the fitness areas endurance is the ability to maintain a pace for an extended period of time. Cardiorespiratory endurance simply means the ability to exercise your entire body without stopping for extended periods of time. Often times this process is simply referred to as cardio. You can slowly increase your cardio endurance over time through exercising that keeps you in your target heart rate for 20-30 minutes. Increasing your cardio can help with your daily tasks such as not becoming tired or out of breath when climbing a flight of stairs, or trying to keep up with your kids. Being in better cardio shape means that you can do anything faster and for a longer period of time, if you find yourself getting out of breath or tired from simple tasks like walking around a store or carrying something up from the basement then maybe you should focus on improving your cardiorespiratory endurance.

Muscular strength is the ability of your muscles to exert enough force to overcome another force such as a barbell. This really just boils down to how strong you are! We mentioned a little about increasing muscular strength through exercise. When you place a stress on your muscles regularly then your body will naturally increase your muscles size and strength. So as you exercise your muscles they will get stronger and over time activities that were once difficult for you to accomplish will become easier. For example if you are curling 15 pound dumbbells and it is difficult for you at first, as you continue to do the exercise over time the 15 pounds will become lighter and lighter to you. This is because your body has adapted to the stress you are putting on it, and you will need to increase the stress to continue improving.

Muscular endurance is the 3rd component of fitness, although it has to do with your muscles it is more closely related to your cardiorespiratory endurance than your muscular strength. Muscular endurance is the ability of your muscles to exert a force repeatedly without becoming fatigued. Think about an exercise like doing sit-ups for a straight minute, it takes a certain amount of abdominal strength but more importantly to sustain the exercise for a minute you need to have muscular endurance or else your muscles will fatigue and you will be unable to continue. Training for muscular endurance helps you to be able to things like repetitive tasks for extended periods of time without tiring.

The forth component of fitness is Flexibility. This is the ability to use your joints and muscles to their full range of motion. At this point in time you might not have great flexibility, but it is something that is never too late to improve. Our muscles are connected to our bones by tendons, and these muscles are used to move joints or stabilize bones. If you do not include flexibility into your routine then your muscles and tendons can become tight. As our muscles tighten up our range of motion can be limited. Tight muscles can also pull on our joints and bones causing discomfort or pain. A good example of this is the association between tight hamstrings and lower back pain. Your hamstrings are the group of muscles that run along the back of your legs, and when they are tight they can pull on your hips and lower back causing your back to ache. Taking a few minutes a day to stretch your hamstrings can help reduce your back pain. Are only a couple of minutes of your time a day worth it for your back to not hurt anymore? I think so!

The final component to fitness is body composition. I am sure you have all seen the BMI weight/height charts; body composition is a more specific version of that. Your body composition is what makes up your physical body; it is the lean tissues and the fat tissues. Lean tissues are all of our muscles, bones, organs and water, while fat tissue is just the fatty tissues of the body. There are several ways to measure this, you can use electrical impedance devices that send a small electrical signal through your body and measures your fat content. You can use skinfold caliper that measures the thickness of the fat under the skin at specific parts of the body, or the simple BMI charts. Your doctor can help you to determine your body composition.

For this week we will be going over each of these components in more detail with specific examples of what type of activities fit each fitness component. Then you can begin to think about what type of activities you would like to participate in to achieve each component.

Now that you have been working on monitoring your portions and calories it is time for you to begin putting what you have learned into practice. By now you have figured out how many calories you need a day through your TDEE, and you know how to count your calories through portion control and reading nutritional labels. So now let's start the weight loss journey, begin by cutting your daily calorie intake by 300 calories per day. So you should consume 300 fewer calories than what your TDEE number is. Keep in mind you will be hungry as your body adjusts to the fewer calories but you will adjust! Remember to count the calories from condiments as well! Dipping fries in ketchup adds calories you need to account for!

Cardiorespiratory Endurance

Improving your cardiorespiratory endurance can feel more difficult than it actually is. If you are like most people you likely have not focused on building your cardio endurance up, or you have very low cardio endurance. The truth is that when it comes to exercise there is a very heavy use it or lose it principle at play. Basically when it comes to your cardio if you have not been training it to improve it then it is going to be low.

The first step in the process of improving your cardio is to admit to yourself that you will have to start slow. You will not be able to move as fast or go as long as you would like to. Admitting this to yourself will help you to not become discouraged. Maybe you can't walk a mile yet, or you can't jog that lap yet. The key word is yet; you need to build up to your bigger goals. Start small and understand that you will have limitations, then over time go a little further or go a little faster. Over time your cardio will improve a great deal, and you will see a big improvement over the course of a few weeks or a month. In fact you won't believe where you will be 6 months or a year from now!

Now we understand what cardiorespiratory endurance is, and that we need to start slow and build it up over time, but what are some of the activities you can do to improve it? You will want to participate in aerobic type of exercises and activities. Aerobic means the requirement of oxygen. Aerobic activities are usually referred to as cardio activities in which you perform moderate to vigorous activity for an extended period of time. As we have learned our bodies use the oxygen in our blood to move and function properly. When participating in cardio activities your cardiorespiratory system needs to be able to meet the oxygen demands of your muscles. If your cardiorespiratory system cannot keep up with the oxygen demands then you will become fatigued and tire out. This is why it is important to go at a pace that you can maintain for an extended period of time, but also strenuous enough to work your cardiorespiratory system hard enough to force improvement.

Some of these types of activities include running, biking, swimming, boxing/kick boxing. Aerobic can be activities like jumping jacks, burpees, circuit training, dancing and so on. The key to this is to find something that you enjoy doing, and then it won't feel like a chore to participate in. You might enjoy going for a light jog after work to clear your head, or maybe you enjoy dancing so you do Zumba or take a dance class. The point is that you can have a variety of activities that you like to do and get a workout in in the process. It is not all running for hours on end! Simply taking 30 minutes to an hour a day could be all it takes to improve your life.

During this week think about the type of activities you enjoy doing and see if you can use them to improve your cardio endurance!

9

Muscle Strength

There are so many misconceptions out there about building your muscle strength. Most people are under the impression that you have to spend hours in the gym lifting heavy weights and chugging protein shakes. Yes, you can gain muscle strength through that type of exercise but that is not the only way! We are going to learn a little more about what types of exercises you can participate in to gain muscle strength, as well as, some of the benefits to building your muscles.

First off building up your muscles can cause an increase in your metabolism. As we have already learned your metabolism is just the process of burning calories for energy in the body. When you increase the size of your muscles then you are increasing the amount of calories it takes to maintain those muscles. This is a big deal; it means that you are able to burn more calories throughout the day even when you are at rest! Increasing the strength of your muscles can help to improve your personal appearance, and reduce your risk of injury during activity. When your muscles are strong it will help to stabilize your joints and could reduce joint pain. You will also be able to pick up heavier objects which depending on your goals could be a big motivator.

Typically the types of exercises that you will engage in when trying to improve your muscular strength are considered anaerobic activities. Anaerobic means without oxygen. So these activities are ones that are explosive, quick, and short lived. This includes things like lifting heavy weights, or sprinting as fast as you can for 100 yards. These activities rely on stored energy in your cells to provide your muscles the energy to function. This stored energy is burnt up very quickly as the pace for the activity is too fast for your cardiorespiratory system to provide the energy. This means that you are not able to maintain this level of activity for a long continuous time.

Now that we know a little about the nature of the activities, what are some examples of exercises you can do? You can lift weights, use resistance bands, climbing stairs/hills, cycling, and body weight exercises. It boils down to any activity that puts resistance against your muscles. This resistance will cause your body to adapt and grow to meet the demand you are placing on it. It is very important to start slow so that you do not overload your muscles and cause pain. Muscle soreness is common but do not use it as an indicator of a good or bad workout.

During this week think about the type of activities you enjoy doing and see if you can use them to improve your muscular strength!

10

Muscle Endurance

As I mentioned in earlier sections muscle endurance is closely tied to cardiorespiratory endurance. There can be a lot of overlap with activities that benefit both your cardio endurance and muscular endurance. Although they are similar they are not the same! Muscular endurance is the ability of your muscles to function at a high level over a period of time. Just having a great cardiorespiratory endurance doesn't mean that all of your muscles are able to function with a high endurance.

Think of it this way, you might be a runner. You run all the time and this has improved your cardio endurance a great deal. Because of the running long distances you have trained your leg muscles to the point that they have high muscular endurance. One day you decide to change your workout up a little and instead of going for a run you decide to jump into the pool and swim some laps. You might notice that you become winded or certain muscles wear out and become fatigued much sooner then when you were just running. This is due to using different muscles in different physical activities. So in this example you might have had great leg muscle endurance but the muscles in the arms do not. So although your cardio endurance was high your arm muscles wore out and became fatigued. As you can see your cardio endurance and muscle endurance are similar but muscle endurance tends to remain specific to the muscles you are training often.

So what are some of these types of activities? I already mentioned 2 possible activities which were running and swimming. You can also participate in cycling, hiking, rock climbing, orienteering, walking, skating, and so on. The idea is to put moderate to vigorous stress on your muscles for extended periods of time. Much like the cardio you need to accept that your muscular endurance might not be great so you will need to start out low and slowly build up as you improve your endurance. Remember you might not be able to do something yet, but you will be there in time. The improvements you can make in a week, a month, 6 months, a year will make you realize how far you have come. When you finish this book you can think back on where you started and really see how much you have grown.

During this week think about the type of activities you enjoy doing and see if you can use them to improve your muscular endurance!

11

Flexibility

This component of fitness is often overlooked, but it is just as important as all of the others! As mentioned earlier, flexibility refers to your ability to use your body's range of motion. What does that actually mean? Well think about your joints, have you noticed that your joints don't move as far as you get older? Have you noticed that it has become more difficult to touch your toes or lifting your leg straight up just doesn't happen easily anymore? If you are experiencing this then your range of motion is becoming limited. Often times I hear people say that they just can't move like they use to or their joints are not what they use to be. The truth is that you can always improve your flexibility no matter how inflexible you might be at this point in time.

The benefits of flexibility were mentioned earlier they are important enough to go over them again. Remember I mentioned how your muscles and tendons can become tight and pull on your joints and bones causing you a great deal of pain. I used the example of stretching out your hamstrings to reduce lower back pain, however stretching out your whole body can help to reduce pain that you might feel in other places as well. Increasing your range of motion can also help you in your day to day lives! Think of all of the movements you need to do all day long, do you think you could do these things better if you could bend at the waist further? Or reach above over your head at the shoulder joint to a greater degree? The truth is that having a greater range of motion can improve your quality of life and performance more than you ever thought. Another added benefit is you could reduce your risk of injury. When your muscles and joints are more flexible then the risk of straining them is reduced. Maybe you are someone who has sprained an ankle in the past. A sprain occurs when the ligaments, which attach bone to bone, have a more than normal stretching force applied to them. This can cause a great deal of pain and swelling as well as take a while for the ankle to heal. Stretching of the ankle can greatly reduce your risk of injury by allowing the ankle joint to have a greater range of motion. This means that with a greater range of motion the joint will be able to move more to accommodate the strain being placed on it. Due to this the likelihood of the joint becoming sprained is reduced!

There are all sorts of stretching and flexibility plans out there that you can pick. Some of them can be calm relaxing stretching while others can be more difficult or focus on strength and endurance building. You can try things like yoga, tai chi, Pilates, or just find a handful of stretches you like and participate in them. It is recommended that you participate in stretching based activities 2 to 3 times a week, but stretching every day would be optimal.

Just like all of the other fitness components you might not be as flexible as you would like to be. You might not be able to touch your toes right now or the range of motion in your shoulders is poor at the moment. The key is to start working on it now and slowly build up overtime. It is important to know that stretching should not hurt; if you are having pain then you are pushing it too far. Start out small and build up to it. Go as far as you can where you can feel the muscles stretching but no discomfort. Hold in that position for 30 seconds and then release. Over a short period of time you will notice how much more flexible you have become. You might notice less aches and pains in your life as a result. For me I like to start my day with a little light stretching then perform a more intense stretching routine later in the day. It is important for you to find what works for you!

During this week think about the type of activities you enjoy doing and see if you can use them to improve your flexibility! Maybe start out small and try to touch your toes. If you can't make it go as far as you can, see how long it takes for you to get to your toes. If you can touch your toes try working toward putting your palms flat of the floor. The key is to strive for small improvements!

12

Body Composition

Body composition is an easy enough concept to understand but it is an important component of fitness when you are looking at obtaining a healthier body and life. As we have gone over already body composition is the comparison of the amount of body fat you have to your lean tissues that include muscle, bones, water and organs. This is a more accurate way of determining the health of your body than the standard BMI number or chart.

I am sure that almost everyone reading this book has had their BMI checked by a doctor at a check-up at some point in your life. Now for the average person a BMI can give a pretty standard measurement for their health and where they should be. However where a BMI check comes up short is that it basically only takes your height and weight into account. In fact that is something that I often hear from people when complaining about their BMI, "I have a lot of muscle so BMI says I am obese but really I am not". Have you heard or told yourself that before? Be honest. The ugly truth is that if you're telling yourself that then you are probably telling yourself a lie. A body composition tests far more than a BMI check, and can give you an accurate representation of how much body fat you have and how much lean muscle you have. It can also provide you with a realistic goal weight to achieve.

People's shapes and sizes can differ greatly from person to person. However 2 people of identical weight, age, and sex can look drastically different. You might see a person you believe is "skinny" who's weight is 185 lbs, and at the same time you might have another person who is an identical weight but you perceive them as being "muscular". The different is body composition. The "skinny" person could be someone who has a low muscle percentage and a higher body fat percentage. This causing them to not appear to be overweight but they could still be holding an unhealthy level of body fat on them. Remember back to what is fat section; visceral fat can be located in the abdominal cavity around the organs. So a person who might be "skinny" could still have a high fat content that could be causing damage to their body despite their outward appearance. Whereas the "muscular" person of equal weight could have a lower percentage of body fat and a higher percentage of lean muscle, giving them a more muscular build at the same weight as the "skinny" example.

There are several methods for finding your body composition levels, some of which your doctor might be able to provide. There are also commercially available products you can use to check your body composition. Some of the most common commercially available items include the electrical impedance devices. These are often seen in handheld devices or house hold scales. How they work is through resistance to electrical signals that are sent from the device through the body. You will not feel the signals but the device measures how long it takes for the signal to be sent out and returned. The signal moves through muscle and fat at different rates and then uses that data to determine your body composition. A doctor might be able to also use skin fold calipers to test the level of body fat you have. This is done by measuring specific areas on your body and plugging them into an equation to determine your body composition. This is a commonly used technique due to the low cost of the equipment. There are also air displacement and water displacement devices. For the air displacement you enter into a pod type device and it measures the amount of air you displace from the device to determine your body composition. The water displacement follows the same principle; however it has fallen out of fashion since it requires a large amount of equipment and can be stressful for the test subject. It is best to discuss your options with your doctor to determine what would be the best option for you.

13

Working out is it Necessary?

I am often asked about different workouts or what people should try when wanting to lose weight. I think that many people believe that without hours of exercise they can't lose weight, and the truth is that you can lose weight without exercise. As we discussed already your weight is controlled by calories consumed vs calories used. So what you eat determines how much body fat you have or do not have, and determines if you are going to gain or lose weight. All of that being said, from what we have learned so far do <u>you</u> believe that working out or exercising during this journey is necessary?

If you want to improve your overall health and quality of life then yes working out and exercise is necessary. We have spent this last week learning about the 5 components of fitness and their effects on the body. We have learned that through exercise we can reduce aches and pains you might experience, we can improve the range of motion of our joints, we can improve the strength of our muscles as well as how long we can use them for. All of this can aid you in reaching your health related goals. There is a reason why you often hear the term diet and exercise in the same sentence; the two go hand in hand.

Since you are here reading this book it is safe to assume that you are ready to make a change in your life. You know that you have issues with your weight and health, and these issues could be affecting your daily life in a number of ways. We have learned that you can reduce your weight and by connection reduce some of the issues associated with your weight through a dietary change. However as you might be starting to discover, just losing the weight is only part of the equation to a life style change. There are a number of benefits to exercising that can improve your quality of life and complement your weight loss in many ways. We will now review some of the ways that adding exercise to your life can result in great changes.

For everyone there is a "toning" effect to increasing your muscular strength, this toning is a tightening of your muscles more or less. Training your muscle strength through resistance training can help to increase your muscle definition and give you a more athletic build. There is also the added effect of increased muscle size results in more calories burnt per day to maintain them, so a boost to your metabolism. Research has also shown that exercise can help to improve your mood and make you feel happier. This is done because exercise can increase the production of endorphins which are known to create positive feelings in the body. Are you someone who has struggled with depression? Research has shown that when a person diagnosed with depression exercises at any intensity they have a significant reduction in feelings of depression, as well as a reduction in anxiety levels.

We have already learned that through exercise we can improve our muscles and bones. Our bodies respond and adapt to the stresses that we place on them. Overtime our bodies will increase in strength and endurance abilities as well as an increase in bone strength through increases in bone density. It might seem counterproductive on paper but exercise can also increase your energy levels! If you are someone who feels tired or has chronic fatigue then adding exercise to your routine can really help to reduce your fatigue levels. You might have heard of this as a runner high. Some of the other benefits include improved quality of sleep, improved memory and information retention as well as reducing your chance of chronic disease and many forms of cancer.

Beyond the impact working out or exercise can have on weight loss there can also be an amazing effect on improving your quality of life. Looking at the list of benefits you can receive from adding exercise to your life, do you see anything on that list that you suffer from? Be honest, do some of the issues you have reside on that list? Ask yourself, would 30 minutes of your day be worth it if it could improve some or all of those issues for you? Does that make working out necessary? I think so.

14

The "I don't have time to exercise" myth

After reading yesterday's section on the benefits of adding exercise to your daily routine you might have come away from it understanding the importance of exercise. However if you are like most people you were having concerns and probably doubts about the amount of time you have available to you, and don't know if your able to fit in exercise to your busy life. After yesterday's reading did you have an internal conflict? Did you tell yourself that you are just too busy to exercise? If you did then you know that you were lying to yourself.

I get it, we fill our lives with various activities and responsibilities and it can be very difficult to add something else to our schedules. The truth is though that you do have the time in your day, you just have to make sure you are allowing yourself to use it properly. I know we have things like work, school, kids, appointments, practices, extracurricular activities we have to take the kids to, laundry, dinner, dishes, and so on. All of those things need to be fit into your day. I know it is tough, I work a full time job, I have a 2 year old son and I am writing this book on top of all of those responsibilities that I mentioned above. Yet despite all of that I still fit in at a minimum of 30 minutes of exercise a day, most days over an hour.

I am able to do this because I prioritize my health and wellbeing. I have occasionally seen on the news and on the internet "fit" parents get demonized for being fit and taking away time from their kids/responsibilities to workout. Think, have you ever had that thought? Have you seen that train of thinking? Have you ever heard someone say something along the lines of "I could be like them, but I would rather spend time with my kids/family instead of being in the gym for hours!" I have heard many versions of that sentence over the years, and I can tell you that it is nothing more than a crutch and a lie people tell to themselves to justify their poor health or weight problems. I stay physically fit for my own health and to set an example for my child. If I fail to take care of my own body then I could be showing my child that they don't need to take care of theirs. At this point in time I can out play my son, I can chase him around the yard, and I can get on the floor and roll around with him. I can be a more engaged father because I take the time to prioritize my health.

I am in no way calling anyone a bad parent, but I am focusing on a lie that I hear repeated often. The truth is that my taking time for myself is as much a benefit to my child as it is to me. I set a healthy example and I reduce the risk of chronic disease/ cancer later in my life. My decisions now could help me to be around for my children for a longer time then if I "let myself go". So do you still find yourself in the "I don't have time" camp? Let's continue then.

According to new information from the Nielson report Americans are consuming an average of almost 6 hours of video per day. That includes watching live TV, DVR styled content, apps, smartphones/tablets, and internet content. That is an enormous amount of time that you might be spending on media. There is a clear shift in the type of media that is being consumed, the younger generation of 18-34 year olds are migrating to digital platforms like Netflix and other online sources. However the result is still the same, a large amount of time is spent viewing some sort of media. We are all guilty of binge watching something, or sitting down and relaxing for a night watching our favorite shows or browsing social media.

At this point you are probably thinking to yourself that you do not watch that much TV! I barely have time to sit during the day! You might be telling the truth to an extent, you very well might not watch that much media or your schedule but that doesn't mean you don't have other vices taking up your time. The key is to prioritize your time and find a way to fit in activity, you might not be able to fit in a large amount of time every day but if you have to make time if you are truly wanting to make a change in your life.

This is where this sections challenge will come in. Remember how I had you begin to count your calories and monitor your portion sizes without making any changes to your dietary choices? We are going to follow the same idea here, because it is important for you to take an objective look at your daily life in order to understand what changes need to be made. For the next week I want you to record your daily schedule, how you do it is up to you. Keep notes on your phone; write down on a note pad, anything that you can keep on your person for the entire day. What you need to do is account for all of your time in the day. So for example you might wake up at 6 am and have to be at work at 8 am. So account for all of the time you used and what you were doing between the time you got up and the time you got to work. Do the same for your work day. Keep track of your commute, how much time you spent on dinner and be precise. Did you come home from work and sit down for an hour or so before you started dinner? Account for all of the minutes of the day and what you are doing; write down what time you started an activity and what time you completed it. For example "started dinner at 5:32, and completed dinner at 6:13" "ate dinner 6:15-6:45" "Began dishes at 7:00" "TV at 7:15-8:45" "kids in bed at 9:05".

Do this practice for a week; you might be surprised how much time you spend on activities like TV, social media, and other tasks. Review your daily schedule closely, you will find a time that you can fit exercise in. I am not asking you to cut out your leisure time, because we all need our downtime. However having too much downtime at the expense of your health is a bad thing. You might find that you can make an adjustment to your morning routine that could save you 20 minutes, and saving that 20 minutes coupled with waking up 15 minutes earlier could give you enough time in your day to exercise! Small adjustments to your schedule could yield big results for your weight loss and health; you just need to find what works for you.

Finding what exercise is right for you

After the last section you might be realizing that in this book there is a certain amount of tough love and a call for self-reflection on your choices that might not always be the easiest thing to swallow. The examples I provided might not always apply to you specifically but that doesn't mean that you do not need to self-assess your own life to make adjustments. The truth is that you are reading this for a reason, and some people need to come to the realization that some of your choices have led you to where you are now. That being said it is time to take a look at other choices that you can make going forward to help you with this life style change. This choice is about what sort of exercise or physical activity is best for you.

We covered the idea of having to make your physical fitness a priority in your life and that you need to ensure that you are applying the appropriate amount of time to your physical health. Now where do we start? Do we run on the treadmill for hours? Do we use that made for TV thing you bought 3 years ago and is still setting in your basement? Do we join a gym? How about taking classes? For some people those choices could be perfect, for others those could be miserable. The key to this section is to learn about what you might enjoy doing so that it feels less like a duty and more like a fun activity.

We are busy, and you should be currently assessing how busy you are in your life. You need to take into account your schedule and how much time you have and when you have it, when picking an activity. For example maybe you have realized that you have an hour in the mornings so you decide to stop at the gym you pass on the way to work. Or you have 35 minutes between the time you get home from work and the time you need to get the kids off the bus, so you take the dog for a long walk. Your exercise needs to fit into your life, so keep that in mind when you are deciding what you would like to do.

You need to pick something that you have the resources available to you. Maybe you enjoyed lifting weights when you were younger and might want to start that up again, so you join a nearby gym. Maybe you have that bike sitting in the garage that you have been meaning to ride, for years. How's that treadmill that has been used as a clothes rack since 2 weeks after you bought it? Do you have a nice walking path available to you? Does your employer have a gym on the premises? Maybe your local YMCA or fitness club offers classes you could take like a spinning class, yoga class, or Zumba type classes. Are there local sports leagues you could check out like a basketball league, softball leagues, or volleyball? The point is to research what is available to you in your area. There are resources online, things like fitness channels on YouTube that provide free content or workouts. Maybe you are someone who can be self-motivated and you can plug in a DVD to a workout program you bought and be fine doing that every day. Maybe you are not self-motivated and struggle when on your own. If that is the case then you need to take that into account and maybe join a fitness class or have a friend exercise with you.

The important thing is that you need to set yourself up for success by knowing what you like and what motivates you. Picking an activity that you hate or putting yourself in an environment that could affect your motivation would be setting yourself up for failure. You can also perform a variety of activities to keep things interesting and to hit on all the 5 components of fitness. Changing up your routine or performing a variety of exercises will help to keep your workouts from getting stale and boring. So you might find that you really enjoy yoga, which is an exercise that can hit several of the components of fitness, and you decide to supplement that workout by running or walking. You might do yoga 4 days a week then run/walk the other 3 days. Maybe in the winter months you do yoga 4 days a week and joined a volleyball league at the YMCA that meets twice a week. The point is that you are not stuck with your choice permanently; you can perform a variety of things. You just need to stay active!

You have to remember that you need to be able to fit it into your schedule. If you chose to do something that doesn't fit into your time frame then you will either not complete it at all or you will regularly miss sessions. It has to all work together, what you like to do and when you have time to do it! Finally you have to have reasonable expectations. If you are someone that hasn't exercised in years or who is obese then maybe you shouldn't joint a rock climbing gym right away. It might be something you would like to do but you have to pick something that you can physically do right now. If what you would really like to do is not a reasonable activity at this time then make it a goal and work towards being able to do that activity.

This sections challenge is to begin researching what you would like to do for exercise. You should be starting to understand where you can fit activity into your schedule, and how much time you have available to you. Now it is time to figure out what you like to do! Do some research, see what is out there. Maybe you already have an idea of what you can do; maybe it has never crossed your mind yet. The important thing is to be honest with yourself; you know what you enjoy doing and what you don't. Take a few days to try somethings out, and don't be afraid to step a little out of your comfort zone! Ignore things like exercise gender norms/stereotypes. Not all men have to love weight lifting, not all women have to do yoga, do what you enjoy and it will be easier to follow through!

16

Hurting your workouts with rewards

It is a common practice for people to feel that they can reward themselves for working out with a treat. Often times that treat is in the form of some type of high calorie junk food or a beverage they know they shouldn't be consuming. But it's ok to eat that thing because you worked out today, right? Wrong. This is a classic form of self-sabotage and if you have this mindset then you are setting yourself up for failure. Rewarding yourself from time to time is not a bad thing, as long as you are accounting for it in your daily caloric needs.

Let's look at a few examples here. Walking a mile will burn roughly 100 calories on the average person. For some people the act of walking a mile will burn more calories than others and vice versus. Now think of something that you might consume as a "reward" for your workout. For some people it might be a Pumpkin Spice Frappuccino from a popular well know coffee house chain. Looking at the nutritional information for the stated drink, in a 16 oz cup there is 450 calories. To put that into perspective you would need to walk around 5 miles just to offset the amount of calories in that single "reward". Ask yourself is it worth it? To put it another way you might have to swim laps vigorously for 45 minutes to an hour or more to work off the calories in that drink!

Rewarding yourself from time to time is an important thing. Cutting out everything you love will make you miserable and want those things all the more. As we have learned though, you need to account for those foods in your daily calorie allowance. If you are regularly rewarding yourself because you worked out then you could be shooting yourself in the foot multiple different ways. First off you might not be burning as many calories in your workout as you think you are. Sure there are apps and devices that you can use that will give you a rough estimate but they are not perfect. You might think you burnt 400 calories during your workout but in reality maybe you only burnt 200. As we have gone over several times now, over eating by an average of only 100 calories can pack on the pounds a significant amount over time. Rewarding yourself because you worked out can cause you to be over eating and undo a lot of the work you have been doing!

Secondly, rewarding yourself is adding unnecessary calories to your daily intake. Adding in these calories means your body has to burn those at some point or turn them into fat. At this point in time you know how many calories you need a day, and you have begun eating fewer calories than your TDEE says you need. This is how you force your body to use fat for fuel. If you are rewarding yourself then you could be reducing the amount of fat your body is using for fuel, which will only make it take longer for you to reach your goal weight. The saying "A moment on the lips, forever on the hips" comes to mind! Pay attention to your habits, allow for the occasional reward but do not make it a regular habit.

17

Life is 7 days a week not 5

Many people see their health and fitness like they see their job, a Monday to Friday 5 day work week. Because of this mindset people tend to take the weekend off of their health and fitness responsibilities. Doing this could cause you to over eat or skip out of physical activity. Your body doesn't stop its processes on Saturday and Sunday and start back up again at 8 am Monday morning, and neither should your healthy life style.

At this point in time you are running in a 300 calorie deficit, this means that you are eating 300 fewer calories than your TDEE says you need to maintain your weight. At the end of this week you will be moving to a 500 calorie deficit and maintaining there for some time. For this example we will be using the 500 calorie deficit for the sake of easy math.

Cutting 500 calories a day from your TDEE means that you are running a deficit of 3500 calories a week. Does that number sound familiar? It should, because that is how many calories are in a single pound of fat. However that number of a weekly deficit of 3500 calories comes from 7 day week. So let's look at it from a 5 day week now. A 500 calorie deficit for 5 days is 2500 calories, a full 1000 calories less. That might not seem like much but how much is that over a period of time? In a time frame of 2 months or 8 weeks that difference of 1000 calories a week adds up to 8000 calories, which is a little over 2 pounds worth of fat you did not lose just because you took the weekends off. Over the period of 6 months that adds up to 24000 calories, or just shy of 7 pounds of fat worth of calories. What about a year? That's 52000 calories, or roughly 15 pounds of fat. Remember we learned that a pound of fat is roughly the size of a standard can of vegetables or soup. So if 15 pounds of fat doesn't sound like much for just taking the weekends off, think of it in terms of volume. Stack 15 cans of soup up on your counter and look at the total amount of space in your body 15 pounds of fat can take up!

All of this is assuming that on your "weekend off" you are only eating up to the calories required in your TDEE to maintain your current weight. If you were to over eat or cheat on the weekends then you could easily be undoing several days' worth of work from the weekdays. You have so far been monitoring the calories in your food; think about how much you could over eat in a weekend by returning to your old habits. Could it undo all of the work that you achieved during the week? Is it worth it? Because of this I recommend that you take all 365 days of the year seriously and do not use the weekends as your reward or cheat days. You just might sabotage all of your progress so far.

18

Your skinny friend is Neat

We have covered so much information in this book so far. The idea is to build up your knowledge on how the body works early on and then apply it. What makes this book different from other weight loss books is that I want to teach you everything that you need to know to make good choices about your health. I do not want to tell you what you can and cannot eat or prescribe specific exercise plans that you have to follow in some get fit quick scam. It is easy when someone in the health and fitness field to assume that their audience knows more than what they really do. Think about what we have covered so far, how much of the information was new to you? I want this to be a different experience for you, where at no point am I ever talking over your head because I have been slowly building up your knowledge base on the subjects. This leads us right into our next topic, which is that your skinny friend that seems to eat whatever they want and never work out and never gain a pound, well they are neat.

As you read earlier there are some hard truths that you might have had to accept about yourself and your mindset towards this journey we are on. Some of them might have been easier than others, and some of the information you might not have accepted yet. One of the most common things I get resistance from people is the information we already covered about metabolism. Ever since that section you might have had it in the back of your head or even have stated it out loud, "If what I told you about metabolisms is correct then why do I have a friend that eats all sorts of junk foods and never exercises but they stay skinny!" Well the fact of the matter is that there does seem to be people like that out there, would you hate me if I told you that people tend to see me that way?

I chose not to cover this subject right after the metabolism section because I wanted to build up more of a knowledge base for you on activity and the effect it has had on the body. I also wanted you to think on the subject for a while, even if you didn't realize that you were. The truth is that there are some people out there that seem to be genetically gifted and can eat and eat and not gain weight, but is there more to this story than what meets the eye?

Your naturally skinny friend is neat. Not neat as in cool but neat as in the acronym N.E.A.T. This stands for Non-exercise activity thermogenesis. This term sounds far more complicated than it really is and it boils down like this. We know that we burn so many calories during the day just to maintain our body systems, this being our BMR. On top of that we know how many calories we burn a day when we add in our exercise levels, this is the TDEE. But what is in-between these two concepts? This is where N.E.A.T comes into play. Non-exercise activity thermogenesis accounts for the calories we burn from things that are not sport like exercises, this can include things like walking to work, performing yard work, walking across the office to the copier, typing, general movements, fidgeting, and so on.

All of our movements require the use of calories as fuel, they do not always require a lot of calories but a little amount adds up quickly. A small experiment was conducted and reported in the BBC News about the effects of standing vs sitting all day (A subject we will touch on more later in this book). The experiment took 10 office workers who sit all day and had them stand for 3 hours a day at work. That sounds like a lot of time spent standing but in reality there are many ways you can do this. General standing, stand when on the phone and so on. They concluded that due to the increase in muscle activation and heart rate that the participants were burning about 50 more calories an hours standing rather than sitting. That doesn't sound like a lot but to put that in perspective if you were to stand at work every day for 3 hours that's 750 calories extra burnt in a 5 day work week. In the course of a year that could add up to around 39,000 calories or just over 11 pounds of fat burnt doing nothing but standing for extra time during your work day.

As I mentioned before fidgeting is something that can burn calories, again maybe not a lot but look at how much the calories added up for 1 year of standing during the workday. Fidgeting can take the form of many habits, foot bouncing, hand gestures while talking, being a "busy body" pacing and so on. As a person who fidgets regularly I could be burning upwards of an extra 200-300 calories a day just with my extra movements that are non-exercise related. So is it that I just have great genetics that allows me to eat a lot and seemly never gain weight or is it because myself and people like me move more often throughout the day and those movements add up.

Apply this idea to information we have already learned. If you over eat by an average of 100 calories a day you will gain around 10 pounds of fat a year. Over 5 years that's 50 pounds, and remember most people put on the weight over several years and not all at once. So let's apply that idea to your friend that never gains weight. They might over eat by the average of 100 calories a day or so but due to their increased N.E.A.T. movements they are burning off those extra calories without having to exercise. This would account for their seemingly unfair food intake and lack of weight gain. You can test this, take note of how often your "naturally skinny" friend really moves; the amount might surprise you and could be the key to their weight maintenance.

Now the truth is that NEAT is not fully understood at this point. We know that the movements that are a part of NEAT burn calories and those calories can add up to be a lot over time. However what we don't know is what controls or regulates our NEAT urges to move. Some research shows that it could be linked to over eating and under eating, this meaning that our bodies will naturally want to move more when we over eat and want to limit movements when we under eat. This concept leads to the idea that spontaneous urges to perform some sort of physical activity could be actually be preprogramed into us as a natural defense against becoming obese.

The time has come for more self-reflection. Look at your habits, do you find that you avoid extra movements even if you don't realize it? Do you find yourself not being willing to cross the room or the office to get something you need or want? Will you take the elevator instead of the stairs even if it's only a single floor? Will you drive around the parking lot looking for the closest spot when out shopping just so you don't have to walk as far? Do you see opportunities in your daily life where you could increase your movements? If so are you willing to make the conscious effort to increase your NEAT? It could make a big difference in your weight loss and your quality of life. All of the little things add up to big long term success.

19

Increasing your NEAT

Now that we have learned that your "naturally skinny" friend might not have better genetics than you and probably just simply moves more throughout the day. That is something that you can consciously change in your life. You can actively make the choice to move more throughout the day. The thing is what can you actually do to increase your NEAT movements? The following paragraphs will put forward some ideas on little things that you can do throughout your day to increase your movements. Some of the ideas will apply to you while others will not. The important thing is that you understand the goal of increasing your NEAT and to adapt the ideas to your life, or to create your own ideas and concepts.

This first one is something that applies to most people regardless of weight or fitness level. How often do you drive around the parking lot of a store until you find a parking spot that is close to the door? Be honest we have all done this, and many of us do it every time we go out somewhere. We do this for a few reasons, first so we don't have to walk as far and 2nd so we don't have to waste time walking from the car to the store. I am a person who generally parks further away, and a few years ago I took note of something. I parked about halfway down the lot and a person who got there before me was driving up and down the rows looking for that perfect spot. As I walked to the store I continued to watch this person drive and drive, until finally I entered the store. So the person driving the car was driving around looking for a spot before I got there and was still searching after I had already entered the store. So it would seem you can waste more time looking for a closer spot then just taking one further down the lot.

I began to think on this some more, and upon leaving the store I decided to count how many steps I took from one parking spot to the next. I found that I take 4 steps from the start of one parking spot to the start of the next. I am a tall guy with a long stride so I am willing to assume that the average person would take about 5 steps for each spot. Why is that important? Well let's say you park at the closest spot in the parking lot that means that you are reducing the number of steps you take by 5 steps per parking spot. Think of it like this, if you parked 30 spots down the lot there is 150 extra steps to the store and 150 steps extra steps on the way back. A very easy way to increase your step totals for a day and increase your NEAT!

How else can you increase your steps for the day? You could take the long ways when at work. So if you are going to a meeting or going to use the restroom at the office walk around the office first then go to your destination. You could take the stairs instead of the elevator. Right now you might be thinking that the stairs hurt your knees to much so you can't do that. You could take the stairs for one floor then ride the elevator the rest of the way, and slowly work on going another floor and another floor over time. Often times when working in an office there can be several different places where printers are located, print to the furthest one away. Go for a walk on your breaks. These are all ways you can get more steps in without wasting much time.

We have already learned that standing burns more calories than sitting. You can try to stand during calls or get a standing desk. When we stand we have to engage several muscle groups to keep us stable and balanced as well as keep us up right. This improves muscular endurance and caloric burn. Try not leaning back in your chair while you work, focusing on good posture will force more muscles to contract to keep you sitting up. General fidgeting can always help as well! Bounce your leg or tap your foot. Have something like a grip squeezer to use while you read things like emails at work. Make it part of your work routine, read emails squeeze the grip strengthener. What's important is to adapt your movements to meet your occupation.

Now what about your home life? Depending on your home life there are several things you can do to increase your neat. When you are done watching TV for the night walk the remotes and place them across the room. This gives you extra steps when you call it a night and when you go to retrieve the remotes later the next day. Make multiple trips when you're bringing in groceries. I know the running joke for everyone is that you would rather die than make 2 trips. However think of all the more time you use making 4-5 trips and how many extra steps you could get in. Clean your house more often. Your house might be spotless or filthy or anywhere in between. If you clean once a week, try cleaning twice a week. Cleaning involves a lot of movements and is a great way to increase your NEAT while also achieving a task! What do you usually do during while watching TV? You usually sit or lay down on the couch, you could try to take 10-20 minutes and stretch during your TV watching. Stretching can be a low effort activity that involves movement and won't interrupt your show!

Now that we know what NEAT is and how much small movements can impact our daily caloric burn as well as some ideas on what we can do to improve our NEAT. Take a couple of days and observe your own habits. Do you always take the elevator? Do you always take the most direct route even though it only saves a minute or two? Once you are consciously observing your own habits you can begin to make the small changes to increase movement. If you work on the 5th floor, take the stairs to the 2nd floor and then the elevator. Stand when on the phone at work or at home. Get an exercise tool that you can keep at your desk like a grip strengthener and use it during easy tasks. Or use it at home during commercial breaks. There are so many small things that you can do that will not inconvenience your daily life but impact your overall health in a bigger way than you can imagine!

20

Setting a Goal

Anytime we want to achieve something it is important to set goals. We have financial goals, personal goals, career goals, school goals, relationship goals, and so on. When you started reading this book and began this journey you probably had a goal in mind. It could be to lose 20 pounds or to lose 200 pounds, maybe you are looking for ways to keep the weight off and that's your goal. No matter what your goal might be the point is that you have one. However, did you create your goal properly? Is your goal going to help or harm your long term success?

The truth about goals is that people don't really know how to make them, or to apply them properly. Take a moment to think about the goal that you wanted to achieve when you started this. If you don't have a goal, take a moment and think of one that is related to the topic of this book. Is your goal vague or specific? Did you set a time frame to achieve your goal? Is it a reasonable goal for you, is it realistic? Is the goal long term or short term? Can it be broken down into smaller goals? These are all things to think about when creating goals, especially one that is as important as your health and weight loss.

There is a template for goal writing that I like to follow, it is known as SMART. As you can see this is another acronym that stands for Specific, Measurable, Achievable, Results focused, and Time. Following this formula you will be able to create goals that you can use to help you along the way, and give you that feeling of accomplishment! Let's start with the S, specific. You need to have some sort of purpose or direction to guide you. Having a specific outcome in mind will allow you to come up with detailed specific plans to reach your goal. You need to know exactly where you want to be so that you can know exactly what you need to do to get there.

The M stands for measurable, which simply means that you need to be able to measure or monitor your progress. This is very important, if what you are trying to accomplish is not measurable in some way then how can you see your progress? Seeing your progress is how you stay motivated! The A stands for Achievable. Your goal has to be realistic to you specifically. You need to be able to see yourself accomplishing your goal. Result focused, the R. This means that you need to focus on achieving results not just completing activity. The final component is Time. You need to set a time frame for when you want to achieve your goal. This could be short term or long term. Short term is something you can achieve in a couple of months or less. Long term can be several months to several years. Be realistic with your time; don't set a goal to lose 100 pounds in 3 months. Set yourself up for success by creating a time frame that will allow you to have enough time to complete your goal but not so much time that you can put it off.

Since you are reading this book your goal is likely going to be weight loss related. Losing weight can take some time to accomplish. You will have times of rapid weight loss followed by times of little to no weight loss, over all weight loss goals are usually long term. For example you might want to lose 150 pounds, so let's start with that. When do you want to lose it by? Is 6 months a realistic time frame? That works out to 25 pounds a month, which might be achievable for the first month or 2 but after that, 25 pounds a month is a lot of weight to lose for an extended period of time. So how about a year? That's

12.5 pounds a month. That seems far more reasonable to lose, however that is still around 3-4 pounds a week that you will have to lose. Let's try for 1.25 years, which is 16 months. That works out to be a little less than 10 pounds a month. That seems like the most realistic amount of weight to lose per month for an extended period of time.

So now we have a goal to lose 150 pounds and a time frame to lose it in which is 16 months. So for an example to make this specific the goal could look like this. "I will lose 150 pounds by May 1st 2019." This is Specific, Measurable, Achievable, Results focused and Timely. However, just because it meets all of the SMART criteria, that doesn't mean that it is any easier for you to attain your goal. 16 months is a long way off, and it can be very hard to stay motivated when you see that 150 pounds you want to lose. What can we do to make this easier?

The goal of losing 150 pounds in 16 months is clearly a long term goal, which means that it can be broken down into smaller more manageable chunks called short term goals. As stated earlier the goal of 150 pounds over 16 months averages out to about 10 pounds a month. So we can take that long term goal and create a short term goal of losing 10 pounds per month. Which looks more attainable losing 10 pounds or losing 150 pounds? Breaking the total weight loss goal down into smaller weight loss goals allows you to achieve a few things. First it provides you with a way to monitor your progress. One month you might lose 12 pounds, and the next you might lose 8, followed by 6 the next month. Monitoring this you can spot trends like a slowing of weight loss, which tells you that you need to make adjustments to your calorie intake. Or you might see that you are consistently meeting your goal of 10 pounds a month on average and know that you need to keep doing what you're doing. Secondly, having short term goals gives you small victories along the way. Using my example 16 months is a long time and it can be easy to lose your way or get disinterested over such a big time frame. Achieving small goals along the way can help to keep you motivated and give you something to strive for in the now.

Take some time to check if your goals are SMART. Look for ways you can break your long term goals into smaller more attainable goals. Set yourself up for success by figuring out what it is you want and when you want to achieve it. Taking the time to create good goals will allow you to set a road map leading you to success.

21

Putting it into Practice

We have been learning all about how to lose weight and how to select the exercises that will work best for your life and your goals. You have been given small tasks to put into practice that include counting your calories, monitoring portion size, looking for ways to increase your daily movements. Now it is time to start putting everything that we have learned into practice.

You should be currently running at a calorie deficit of 300 calories below your TDEE a day. It is time to increase your calorie deficit to 500 calories a day. As we covered earlier, running a 500 calorie a day deficit will put you on pace to lose 1 pound of fat a week. This doesn't sound like a lot but it is a great way to start. Cutting to much out too quickly could leave you feeling very hungry, tired/lethargic, irritable, and just plain miserable. Starting out slowly and building up allows your body to adjust to your new life style. Allowing your body to slowly adjust will increase the likelihood of you sticking with it. The same concept can be applied to becoming more active and engaging in exercising.

When you first begin exercising it is important to not overdue it right at the start. It is very common for your muscles to be very sore for a day or several days following the start of activity. This is just something that you will have to deal with, but you can reduce the muscle soreness by easing into the activity. After some time you will no longer get sore even after vigorous activity. Overdoing it can cause you to become discouraged and quit the activity or miss several days waiting for the soreness to leave your muscles. This can cause setbacks or delay progress.

At this time you have a base knowledge on what you need to do. You have your goals in mind and your physical activities picked out. Today is the day that you begin to put it all in action! We have been slowly building to this day, and we are now 3 weeks in to this journey. This is where the hard work begins; maintaining a daily schedule of working out and eating right is not always going to be easy. You will have set backs and you will have days that you don't want to do this anymore or want a day off. On those days you need to remember why you are doing this, why you decided to pick up this book and start reading. I am not there to hold you accountable, you will have to self-monitor and make the correct choices when it comes to your exercise and diet. Whether you succeed or fail will be on you. Just remember that failure is just a new starting line. Keep reading and applying what you have learned to your life. By the time you finish this book you will be amazed at how far you have come!

22

The importance of your before and after pictures

We have all seen those amazing before and after pictures on various infomercials, on the news or from friends and family on Facebook. We will be covering the truth about those miracle before and after commercials later in this book. For this section we will be taking a brief moment to discuss the importance of before and after pictures for your own personal use.

When you started this book you might have had a particular goal in mind, maybe you just want to become healthier or you want to fit into a certain outfit or those old jeans of yours. No matter what your goal, it can be very difficult to notice the change in yourself while moving towards that goal. So how can you tell that you are making gains in this journey? You can keep track on the scale, you can take measurements, you can feel your pants getting loose, but for most of us seeing results in ourselves is the biggest motivator. There is a problem with this for most of us though, most people do not see the changes in themselves as quickly as they would like. How often have you or someone you know lose some weight and have been told "you look great" or "I can see you lost weight." Only to hear the response "I don't see it yet".

The truth is that that for most people you will be the last to notice weight loss in yourself. It is a matter of perspective, you see yourself every day so small changes go unnoticed. To others who do not see you as often these small changes add up and become more noticeable. Due to this it can become very discouraging for you, because you are putting in all of this effort and not "seeing" the results. Think of it this way, if someone came into your house every day and moved your couch a half inch in the same direction it might take a long time before you notice the change, even though it is there. You see that couch every day and the change is small, so you might not take notice of the change until it becomes a big change from its original position.

Taking a few "before" pictures when you start this weight loss journey will let you see what you looked like when you began. It will give you a comparison to see just how far you have really come, and allow you to be able to refer back to when you need motivation. Don't underestimate the importance of "seeing" your changes, we are still early in this journey and your motivation is probably high but in the coming months you might find yourself losing motivation. Looking at your "before" pictures could help to keep you on track.

23

Starvation Mode Myth

As I am sure you are well aware, there are countless myths and "facts" about weight loss. These myths can range from you shouldn't ever lose weight to the only way to lose weight is by doing xyz and everywhere in between. One of the ones that you might have heard is the myth of starvation mode. Let's review what the starvation mode myth is.

The idea is simple if you cut your calorie intake to much then your body will freak out and slow your metabolism down so much that you won't lose any weight. So let's begin with the thing that is cited most commonly as proof that starvation mode is real, the Minnesota Starvation Experiment. The experiment took military men in 1945 and cut their caloric intake by 55% which means they were eating less than half of what their daily caloric needs to maintain weight (TDEE) was. This is an enormous cut in calories, to put it in perspective most calorie cut recommendations are in the 15 to 25 percent range. For the experiments participants this meant that they were going from about 3,400 calories a day down to 1,500 calories a day. This 1,500 number becomes important with the myth.

The results were basically as expected and did not show that the participants entered into a "starvation mode" and stopped losing weight. In fact the average total weight loss for the participants was a loss of 25% of the original starting weight. On top of the weight loss the participants saw on average a drop down to only having 5% body fat. You might be asking yourself if this is the case then why is the study held up as "proof" of starvation mode. The study did show a reduction in metabolic rate, and as we have learned metabolism is just the process of burning calories. So the study did show that the participants had a reduction in their metabolism burning calories during the experiment of about 40%. So starvation mode must be true, correct? Not exactly, we need to look closer at the results! 25% of that reduction was due to the weight loss itself, remember back to when were learned about metabolism and BMR/TDEE. The bigger you are the more calories you need to burn to maintain at that size. So when you lose weight you do not need as many calories to maintain a smaller weight, so your metabolism "slows" because you do not require as many calories. What do you think accounts for the remaining 15% reduction in metabolic rate? Here is a hint, NEAT.

Remember when we covered NEAT, your non-exercise activity thermogenesis is linked to your food intake. So when you eat more you subconsciously fidget and move around more, and when you don't eat as much you naturally do not move as much. Your body is complex and smart; when you are in an extreme calorie deficit your body will basically prioritize and will subconsciously reduce your NEAT. Choosing, instead to conserve energy to be used in keeping the major body systems running. Once the participants returned to their normal caloric intake, that 15% reduction in metabolic rate would return to normal. While the other 25% would not return without a gain to the original starting weight. Now it is also important to note that the participants did not experience the reduction in metabolic rate/NEAT until they dropped down to 5% body fat, which is a level that is very difficult to reach.

The results of this study have often times been misrepresented to push this idea that cutting calories is bad and will actually make you gain weight. Remember I mentioned that 1,500 calories a day number was important to the myth? Often when the starvation mode myth is being pushed it is being stated that 1500 calories a day is to low and you will be in starvation mode, because that's what the participants ate! The truth is that 1,500 calories a day was very low for the participants but it was not able to put them into this mythical state where their bodies will not lose weight. For the participants the 1500 calories a day was only 45% of their TDEE, and for the average person you should never cut down that far. It is usually recommended that you only cut 15-25 percent of your total calorie needs. So let's say that your TDEE is 2,000 calories, a reduction of 25% would put you at consuming 1,500 calories a day. Although that is the same total calories eaten a day as the experiments participants that doesn't mean you would be in as large of a calorie deficit. In order to match the participants you would have to cut 55% of 2,000 calories which would mean you would only be consuming 900 calories a day. See the difference? Since every ones TDEE is unique to them the amount of calories consumed to remain in a safe calorie deficit is different. For some 1,500 calories a day is way too low where for others it is just right. Right now you are at a 500 calorie a day deficit, which means you are eating 500 calories under your TDEE. You can now choose to change that up by selecting a calorie deficit in the 15-25 percent range.

Now all of that being said, why does the myth keep spreading? Well there are a few reasons that might keep it going. First weight loss is not always an exact science when it comes to calories cut vs weight on the scale. For example you might be running at a calorie deficit that puts you on track to lose 5 pounds this month, then you step on the scale and you only lost a pound. This could be because you underestimated your caloric intake or you're on a temporary plateau caused by water retention. It is easier to blame something like "starvation mode" than to think that you might have screwed up your calorie counting. Another factor is that many people do not like counting calories, it takes effort and some days it can be unpleasant to have to restrict how much you consume. So it is easier to believe the myth so that you have a reason to not count calories. Finally the diet industry is a very large very profitable beast. The industry makes money off of convincing people they can't lose weight without the help of a product or medication that is being sold.

To recap this, starvation mode is the idea that if you cut calories your body will slow down your metabolism so that you actually won't lose any weight anymore. The truth is that this is simply not true. Although you will see a reduction in your metabolic rate due to your weight loss, this is caused by the amount of weight you lost. When you do not weight as much you do not need as many calories to maintain that size, so it is not that you metabolism is slowing down its more adjusting to your new weight. We have also learned that your NEAT movements could be subconsciously linked to the amount of calories you consume. So reducing your caloric intake could cause you to reduce your NEAT movements.

Now you are in control of deciding how much of a calorie deficit to run per day. You know how many calories are in a pound of fat, you know how many calories you need to maintain at your current weight, and now you know what percent of your TDEE you should be cutting. It is time for you to find what the best fit to reach your goals is. Remember to keep the caloric deficit in a 15-25 percent of your total TDEE range. To find this number simply take your TDEE number and multiply it by the percentage you want to cut. Then take that number and subtract it from your TDEE, this will give you your daily calorie goal.

Exercise: How to do a push up

Being a Health and PE teacher I come across people who don't truly know how to perform certain exercises. So I believe it is important to take the occasional section to go over some of the basic exercises and build up to more complex ones. Up first is the classic push-up.

Although the push up is mostly considered to be a chest and arm exercise it actually benefits the entire body. The primary movers of the push up (which muscles do the movements) are the chest muscles known as the pectorals and the triceps, which are the muscles on the back of your upper arm. However due to the position your body is in to complete a push up many of your other muscle groups play a stabilization role. This stabilization is also known as an isometric contraction. Your muscles of the back, abdomen, and legs all tighten up to keep the body in a rigid form and to maintain balance. While your chest and arm muscles perform movements to lower the body to the floor and raise the body back up to the starting position. But how do we do a push up properly?

For the standard push up you will want to begin in a "Plank" position. This is where your hands are placed on the ground out in front of your body just below the shoulder line. Then your back and legs form a straight line down to your ankles. The other point of contact on to the ground comes at the balls of your feet. So you are balancing your body weight equally between your hands and the balls of your feet. Make sure that your body is in a straight line, do not let your butt and hips sag down or point your butt up in the air. Keeping your body in a straight line will engage your core muscles more, providing more of a workout, and reduce your risk of injury. You want your hands to be placed a little wider than shoulder width apart with your hands in a neutral or slight inward position. Be sure that your hands are below your shoulder line at about your nipple line, this ensures that you will be lowering and pushing yourself back up in a straight motion and not pressing at an angle that can strain your shoulders.

You are now ready to perform the push-up. Lower yourself down taking about 2 seconds to perform the action. You want to lower down to at least a 90 degree bend in your elbows. You can go lower until you are just slightly above the ground when you become more confident in the exercise. Come to a complete stop then press against the ground and raise yourself back up until your arms are fully extended again. This action should be nice and controlled, take about 1 second to perform the up portion of the push up. Going too fast or aggressive on the way up could cause injury to your elbows, while going too fast on the way down could cause you to slam into the ground. Repeat for as many repetitions and sets as you feel you are capable of doing.

As stated above the push-up is a great exercise that you can use to work out your whole body. On top of that you do not need any equipment for it, and it can be done relatively quickly at any point in the day. It is a great exercise for building up muscular strength and muscle endurance. The push-up can also be easily modified so that if you are not able to do a push up at this point in time you can quickly build up to it. So what are some of these modifications?

If you are finding it difficult to do push-ups you can try some variations to make them a little easier. The first variation is the most common one, the knees push up. This is exactly what it sounds like, you will get yourself in the same basic position but instead of the second point of contact with the ground being the balls of your feet it will be your knees. Because you will be on your knees the angle of your push-up will be changed, to compensate for this you may need to adjust the height of your hand placement. This means you might need to place your hands at or above your shoulder line. Over time you will build up your strength and these will become easier for you to complete, as this happens you can keep moving your knees further and further back and then eventually work up to being on the balls of your feet. This might take some time but you will get there.

The next variation is the wall push-up. This is the easier of the two variations listed here. You will be in the same basic position for a regular push-up but instead of having your hands on the ground you will place them on the wall. Then have your feet on the floor out from the wall far enough that you can have your arms completely extended, you will be leaning forward. Lower yourself towards the wall then press yourself back up to the starting position. As you become stronger you can increase the distance your feet are from the wall, and overtime you will build the strength needed to complete a standard push-up. When you are doing a wall push up be sure to have good footing because slipping can be a safety concern.

Push-ups are a great exercise you can add to your daily routine to improve your muscle strength and endurance while also taking up minimal time. Challenge yourself to completing pushups every day. Start with a number that you are comfortable with, it could be 1, or it could be 30. Maybe you can only do 5 at a time, so you decide to do 5 sets of 5 every morning when you get out of bed. Once those become easy add some more, then add some more when that gets easy. Before you know it you will be doing way more than you ever thought you could! Just be sure to breathe while you do them! Often people hold their breath while exercising, inhale while you lower yourself down and exhale while you press back up! Remember a small increase in your daily movement can lead to big improvements in your weight loss.

25

Step Trackers: 10,000 steps a day

Wearable technology is everywhere now, with the advancement it smart phones and internet connections being almost everywhere these days wearable technology that is designed to aid in your fitness is all the rage. I have a Fitbit that I like to use to measure my heart rate and count my steps for me; my phone also has a step counter in it. (I am not sponsored by any company and I am not recommending any specific device, only stating which device I happen to have.) It is common for these devices to come with a daily step goal, most being 10,000 steps a day. Is this a reasonable goal though? Will it help you to improve your fitness?

The short answer is yes. We know that any amount of movement can increase your caloric burn for the day and therefor help you to lose weight, but is 10,000 steps a day to much? Too little? The idea behind the 10,000 steps a day is that it is roughly 5 miles a day, and for an average person of average weight that works out to 500 calories burnt a day just from walking. We already learned that 500 calories cut a day over a 7 day week is 3,500 calories burnt or 1 pound of fat loss. The truth is though that everyone is different and calories burnt can be heavily based on the body weight of the person doing the exercise. Think about it, it takes a lot more effort to move 300 pounds a mile than it does to move 150 pounds a mile. So someone weighing 300 pounds would burn more calories walking a mile than a person weighting 150 pounds, more effort equals more calories burnt.

Now are 10,000 steps to much to expect out of a person? Maybe at first, studies have shown that the average

American takes around 4-5,000 steps a day. That is well short of the 10,000 step goal that most activity trackers set for you. For a sedentary person or for someone who is just starting to become more active you might not be able to reach those 10,000 steps a day. However it is a great goal to strive for as well as a great way to consciously increase your NEAT. Slapping on a Fitbit you might be surprised how few steps you really take a day, so you might have to make a goal to reach those 10,000 steps a day. On top of that you might need to set yourself up to take more steps. I mentioned some strategies for that in an earlier section, park further away, take the long way through the office and so on. If you are not reaching your 10,000 steps a day try increasing your steps by 500 a day every week until you get there.

If you don't have an activity tracker you can still set yourself up to take more steps. Use the methods I mentioned above, take walks more often, and make it a priority in your life to walk more and you will see your step count go up and your weight go down!

26

Aerobic

As you continue to work your way through this journey I am sure that you will be out researching things on your own. You might be looking into different food choices, and making selections based on what you are reading from other sources. You might be reading up on different exercises or workouts you might enjoy. I fully encourage this behavior, but you might be running into the very problem that is the main reason for me writing this book. There is so much information out there and it is easy for the creators of that information to assume that you know more on the topic than what you do. This miss communication can lead to confusion, frustration, and maybe self-injury. As stated before I want to provide you with as much baseline information and build on it that by the end of this book you know enough to take your health and fitness into your own hands. To do this I will introduce concepts throughout these pages that you might come across throughout this process, the concept we are covering today is Aerobic.

What is Aerobic? The simple definition is that it means "with oxygen". Ok, on the surface that doesn't really explain what the term means when it comes to health and fitness. We covered this process very briefly in the cardiorespiratory endurance section, and now we are going to go into greater detail. All of our movements require oxygen, so naturally as we move more during activity we start to breathe heavier and faster to meet the oxygen needs of our bodies. This process is known as our aerobic metabolism. During Aerobic activity our bodies are able to process the oxygen we breathe in and distribute it to where it needs to be at the same rate or faster than our bodies are using the oxygen. This means there is a pace or speed at which you can perform an activity for an extended period of time without fatiguing.

Now that we know what aerobic is, what kind of physical activities are aerobic in nature? These activities are ones that you are able to do for an extended period of time. The most basic example of this is jogging. At this point in time you might not be able to jog at a high pace for a long time, however there is a certain pace that you can jog at that you can hold for an extended periods of time. That pace might be fast or slow, everyone is different and you can increase your aerobic metabolism over time. It is commonly recommended for people with the goal of weight loss to exercise through the use of aerobic exercise.

What happens when we exercise at a rate that causes our bodies to require more oxygen than we can process? When this happens our muscles will become fatigued and tire out, this process is known as the metabolic threshold. When your muscles are consuming more oxygen than your body can produce you will tire out, it is that simple. That being said there is a system in place to keep our bodies going when we cross the metabolic threshold!

27

Anaerobic

As we learned yesterday our bodies have a set point at which we can exercise for extended periods of time without tiring out, but what happens when we exercise at a point that is faster than that point? When we cross the metabolic threshold our bodies will switch from the process of aerobic to the process of Anaerobic. If aerobic means with oxygen what do you think Anaerobic means? By definition anaerobic is "without oxygen".

Anaerobic activities are ones that we can do for a short amount of time before we become fatigued. Think of activities that require quick short bursts of power such as sprinting or weight lifting. When you see someone sprinting in the 100 meter dash their bodies are using energy and oxygen faster than their bodies can supply it. Their muscles will also produce the waste product carbon dioxide faster than they can expel it. So if anaerobic activities do not use oxygen for energy production what is used?

When we exercise at a rate that pushes us past the metabolic threshold our muscles will use the process called glycolysis to produce energy. This is simply the process of our cells breaking down glucose for a quick burst of energy. This process of breaking down glucose, which is just a simple sugar, provides a quick short lived boost in energy but the process also produces lactic acid. This by product serves no purpose to aid in exercise; in fact it will hinder you. Lactic acid will cause your muscles to fatigue and could even lead to muscle soreness.

Sounds like you might want to avoid anaerobic activities doesn't it? Well no, there are benefits to making anaerobic activities part of your routine. Doing activities such as resistance training (think lifting weights) can increase bone density which can reduce your risk of osteoporosis. You can train to increase your lactic threshold, which is the level at which you can handle lactic acid without feeling fatigued. Put simply you can perform at a high intensity for longer. You will also see a boost in energy as your body begins to store more glycogen for energy use. There are also many other benefits to participating regular anaerobic activity.

Taking what you have learned the past two days you will be able to better understand how our bodies respond to specific types of intensities when it comes to exercising. You will come across many different opinions on why one is better than the other and why you should do this instead of that. The important thing I want you to take away from this is that you need to find what works best for you and what you enjoy. If you don't enjoy what you're doing than you're not going to continue doing it. That being said I encourage you to incorporate a little of anaerobic and aerobic activities into your routine!

28

The Importance of Sleep

We all know that sleep is important. Getting your 8 hours of sleep a night is something that we have been told is very important our entire lives! Knowing that, I don't want to turn this section into a lecture boring you by telling you something that you already know. I hope to keep this brief and just go over some of the consequences of not getting enough sleep.

The truth is that many of us do attempt to get enough sleep, but there are things that can cause you to lose out on much needed sleep. You might work night shift and have a hard time sleeping during the day, maybe you have a young child that doesn't sleep through the night. No matter what the cause of your loss of sleep is the important thing is to do your best to try to get enough sleep. What happens if you don't get enough sleep both in the short term and in the long term?

In the short term your sleepy brain might lead you to making bad decisions. What kind of bad decisions? Well, when your sleepy the activity in your frontal lobe dulls and this is an important part of your brain, it controls decision making and impulse controls. See where that can become a problem when you are trying to lose weight? If you are sleepy you could be making it more difficult for yourself to control your portions when eating. Let's face it, when you're tired doing extra activities like working out or exercising can get dropped down the priorities list. Add in reduced decision making skills from a tired frontal lobe and you might be choosing to skip out on your workout for the day. We are not perfect; we all miss workouts or screw up our portion control from time to time. Doing this can cause short term setbacks, but if you limit their regularity then you will still succeed.

However in the long term failure to regularly get enough sleep you might miss workouts often, or fail to maintain your portions several times a week. This will lead to inevitable failure on this weight loss journey. Research has also shown that people who fail to get enough sleep will cause hormonal changes in their body that can effect dietary decisions and weight management systems. Studies have found that people on calorie deficits that were cut back on sleep saw a 55% drop in weight loss from fat. The participants felt hungrier and less satisfied following meals. This can lead you to over eating and feelings of depression or that you have no energy.

I hope reading just those few examples on the effects of not getting enough sleep can have on our weight management shows you the importance of it. Next time you are tired and having the impulse to skip a workout or to eat something or more than you know you should think to yourself "Is this just because I am tired". Doing this might help you persevere!

29

The Effects of Obesity on the Body

Continuing today with things that we all have heard about for years, today we will talk about the effects that obesity can have on the body. Why am I covering this information when I just said that we have all been hearing about this subject for years? My reasoning boils down to two concepts. First being that I am seeking to inform my readers with all of the information that I can, starting with the basics and building up. The second is to give you something to think about when you might be feeling like your motivation to keep going is low. I intend to cover several of the negative effects that obesity can have on your body one by one. Trying to cover them all in one section would cause this single section to become bloated and very long. So the effects of obesity will be sprinkled throughout this book, this section we will be covering type 2 diabetes.

Diabetes is a problem when your body's blood sugar levels rise higher than normal. This condition is known as hyperglycemia and the most common form of this is known as type 2 diabetes. Type 2 is when your body is unable to use insulin in the correct way; you might have heard this before as being insulin resistant. At the start of the disease the body will try to increase its natural insulin produced in the pancreas to make up for it. Eventually overtime your pancreas will not be able to produce enough insulin to keep your blood sugars in a normal range. Insulin is a hormone that allows our bodies to use sugar from carbohydrates from the foods that we eat for energy. It is used by our bodies to keep our blood sugar from getting to high.

Increased blood sugar levels can cause several complications throughout the body. It can damage your eyes, nerves, kidneys, double your risk of stroke and heart attacks as well as cause sexual problems. Eventually it can cause your insulin producing cells in your pancreas to shut down and no longer produce the hormone. This will lead a person to become dependent on outside sources of insulin, known as being insulin dependent and is more common with type 1 diabetics. The problems caused by type 2 diabetes can greatly affect your quality of life, but what is the cause? There is a certain amount of genetics involved with diabetes; however some of the main contributors are being overweight, poor diets, and a sedentary life style. Does that sound familiar?

Now we know what can cause type 2 diabetes and we know what it can do to our bodies. How do we prevent it? By this point in the book I am sure that you are very much aware of what I am going to say! "Lose weight; eat heathier, exercise, and so on". Well if you thought that then you would be correct, but we are going to take a little closer look on just how much you can reduce your risk of type 2 by doing exactly those things. Losing just 7 to 10 percent of your body weight can cut your chances of contracting type 2 diabetes in half! Does 10 percent sound like a lot of weight to lose? It is 1/10th of your body after all. Let's do the math! For example let's say you're a female that weighs 280 pounds. Cutting your body weight by 10 percent would equal 28 pounds. So just losing 28 pounds of body fat could be all it takes to lower your risk of diabetes by half, which sounds worth it to me. Keep this in mind though; according to Harvard an obese person is 20 to 40 times more likely to develop type 2 diabetes than a person of a normal healthy weight. So even though cutting your weight by

10 percent significantly lowers your risk, achieving a healthy weight is your best chance to avoid type 2.

Changing up our diets can also affect our probability of getting type 2 diabetes. Studies show that those who eat an average of 2 servings of whole grain foods a day had a decreased chance of getting diabetes by 21 percent when compared to those who eat refined carbohydrates. What we decide to drink can also greatly influence our risk. Drinking high in sugar drinks such as fruit juices and soda could increase your chances by 31 percent. My final point mentioned was to be more active and exercise, and as you might have guessed being more active will also reduce your risks but by how much? The answer is a whopping 33% or 1/3rd.

The truth is that many of these percentages and risk factors have probably already been mentioned to you either through personal research, other health books, and your doctor or through various other Medias. Maybe these stats have hit home for you before and that's the reason you picked up this book, maybe reading them now with the knowledge you have gained in these pages so far has driven them home for you now, or maybe at this point it still doesn't seem like a big deal to you because your blood work at your last checkup still shows you're fine. If you fall in the last group I mentioned I want you to think of it this way. If type 2 diabetes was a betting game in Las Vegas, who would you place all of your money on? Would you bet on the person who is active, and strives to maintain a healthy weight and diet? Or would you put your money on the person who is overweight or obese with a poor diet and a sedentary life style? All of the percentages and figures we reviewed in this section tell you to place your bet on the second individual doesn't it? So now think, would you place that bet on yourself?

30

Congratulations you have made it through your first month!

Making it a month is a big deal! You should be proud of yourself to have made it this far! We still have a long way to go in this but that doesn't mean that we can't take a moment to pat ourselves on the back. Take today to really reflect on how much we have really gone through this month. You have learned about nutrition, exercise, portion control, the importance of things like sleep, how to perform certain exercises, and finally you have built an understanding of key terms and concepts! You have adjusted your diets, and implemented physical activities into your lives; you are well on your way to creating habits that will lead you to success like you have never seen before. Now with all of that being said some of you might be feeling great, others might be thinking that this past month was very difficult. This is not always going to be easy, but this will also not always be hard.

According to current research it is believed that changes take about 66 days to become habits. So we are about halfway to your new life style becoming second nature. By the end of the next month the things you might be struggling to maintain now will just be something you do without thought! This process takes time and if you allow for that time you will be setting yourself up for success! Today's section will not be covering a new topic, instead it will be a testimony from a person close to me that has made the life style changes and has found tremendous success. Please read through his words, some of what he has to say might relate to you or give you the motivation to keep going.

Losing a significant amount of weight (115# thus far) at 50 years old is very satisfying; however, I certainly wish I had the right drive / motivation to do it earlier in life. Yes, for some battling weight is a lifetime battle but it certainly is not one that you just have to succumb to because of your DNA. It is a battle that can be won with good choices and without surgery. The worst thing that can and does happen to someone that is overweight is acceptance. Don't misunderstand, you must accept who you are as a person and have confidence in who you are; however, you don't have to accept that fact that you are obese. Once you have accepted the fact that you are obese than the obesity has won. It usually starts out as a defense mechanism but once it truly turns into acceptance then defeat is at hand.

Every person battling weight loss has tried nearly every fad diet and gimmick out there; that is why it is a billion dollar industry. But the fact of the matter is most don't work over the long haul as they are not sustainable. Losing weight is about making good long term choices. I enjoy food. I enjoy all types of food. I enjoy food in moderation now. For the most part I have cut sweets / sugars from my diet; however, if I want a cookie I will eat a cookie. I won't eat a dozen cookies or even 6 cookies. I'll eat a cookie. After 6 months of limited to no sugar my body really doesn't desire sugar now anyway. And I was the typical fat kid that loved cake. For me, losing weight has been broken down to simple math. I am simply burning more calories on a daily basis than I am consuming. I do cardio in the form of walking on a treadmill for an hour in the morning (before work) and an hour in the evening (after work). After each treadmill session I have a lifting routine that varies daily based on the muscle group that I am targeting on that day. It is all about finding the right motivation, the right drive. I never thought I would be the person that would do time on a treadmill. Now I do 2 sessions a day. I never thought I would be the person to work out before going to work – that is now my preferred time to work out.

So what is the secret to success? I certainly don't claim any success yet as I am not at my goal; however, you have to be realistic in your expectations and celebrate your successes (mentally more than with pizzas) and surround yourself with encouraging people. Starting on the treadmill I celebrated when I could do just 1 mile at a decent pace with just a 3.0 incline. Then I worked on going just a little bit further every day, just a little bit faster with just a little bit more incline. The first time the treadmill timed out on me at Planet Fitness at 60 minutes I thought the thing broke – I never thought I would spend an hour on a treadmill in one session. At one time I was never able to. When I started out I wanted to lose 10#. After I lost 10 my next goal was 20# and so forth. If I started out with a goal of 100# I would have seen it as overwhelming and probably would have given up after a month. Even now with 115# lost I am focusing on getting to 120# lost. I want each step to be achievable. My weight loss was pretty rapid as I starting in Late March 2018. Speed of weight loss was and is not my goal. Steady progress is. I am satisfied with slow steady progress. I think when I was younger, more immature, if I couldn't get the results right away then it wasn't worth doing – I wish I would have had the long term mind set when I was younger.

I wish I would have known sooner in life that this was possible. I wish I would have known sooner how much better I would have felt if I exercised and took off the excess weight earlier in life. The fact that I don't have knee pain is a wonderful feeling. Waking up with knee pain, for no apparent reason (other than being overweight) was terrible, it was an awful feeling). As you age being overweight seems to be a lot like being in quicksand. The longer you don't do anything about it, the easier it is not to do anything about it, then the more you just get sucked in and the harder it becomes to do anything about it. I wish I would have known sooner that if I really wanted to I could have found the time to get the exercise in that I needed to in order to lose weight.

I hope that after you have read that short testimony his words will be enough to help those who might still be struggling to pick this book up every day and keep reading and apply what you learn to your life. For those of you who have been finding success and not as much struggle I want you to realize that in the near future you could be the one writing to someone about your success and your revelations. We are a month in and have 5 to go, I hope you keep picking up this book and changing your life one day at a time.

31

Exercise: Mountain Climbers

We are going to start out the first day of the new month with a new exercise that you can do without any equipment. The "Mountain Climber" is similar to the push up in the sense that it is a great bodyweight exercise, meaning that it requires no equipment, which engages the whole body. The major difference between the mountain climber and the push up is that when performing a mountain climber your arms remain stationary and your legs do the movements. This exercise is a great cardio exercise and focuses on the lower body muscles.

So what does it look like? Well the starting and ending position looks identical to the starting "up" position of the push up. You want to have your hands placed flat on the floor at about shoulder height and arms fully extended. Keep your core muscles of the abdominals and back tight so that you're keeping your back straight. Just like the push up you want your body to be in a straight line from your head to your toes. You will be up on the balls of your feet so that your points of contact with the ground are the palms of your hands and the balls of your feet.

Now you are in the basic form to begin the exercise. Starting with your right leg you will drive your right knee up to your chest and let your toes make contact with the ground to keep yourself balanced if you need to. Once your right knee has reached your chest begin to lower your right leg to the starting position while at the same time driving your left knee up to your chest. There is a certain rhythm that you will find and the motions will be similar to jogging as you drive one knee up to your chest while simultaneously lowering the other leg back to the starting position and repeat. The object of the mountain climber is to oscillate driving and lowering each knee in rapid succession. This will engage the muscles of the lower body as well as elevate your heart rate.

Keep in mind much like all exercises you might need to start slow and build up to be able to do the mountain climber properly. This exercise will work all of your muscle groups and you might have difficulty holding yourself in the correct position. If this is the first time you are trying this exercise then you should get yourself in the starting position and practice driving each knee to your chest and returning to the starting position before driving the second knee. This will allow you to find your balance and reduce your risk of injury. As you become more confident in the exercise you can increase your pace and the duration of the activity. To start try to do the mountain climber for 30 seconds every day. Once you are able to continuously perform the exercise for 30 seconds keep adding 15 seconds to the time. You will see you muscles become stronger and increase in their muscular endurance. You will get the benefits of improving your cardiorespiratory endurance as well.

32

Spotting Quackery

I once had a professor in college who at the time I thought was a little kooky and was maybe just coasting into retirement enjoying his tenure. He would spend a great deal of time covering the topic of quackery, which to a 21 year old college student who was studying to be a Health and PE teacher it seemed like a no brainer topic. Having been out of college for several years and working in the health and fitness field I now realize that I was wrong. To someone who is just entering the field, quackery seemed like a "no brainer why are we wasting our time on this subject". The truth is that looking back I realize that although he might have been a little kooky, that professor knew that there is an enormous billion dollar industry built on people's inability to spot quackery. That is why the topic of quackery is finding itself covered at this point in time in this book. You might be looking at certain products to aid you in this weight loss and fitness journey but do you know how to spot the difference between something useful or something that's just quackery?

From the context clues in the intro to this section you might have been able to draw your own conclusions on what quackery is, let's start with the definition. Quackery is "dishonest practices and claims to have special knowledge and skill in some field, typically medicine." So basically quackery when it relates to the health and fitness areas is when someone or something makes claims about how to best lose weight or get in shape. Now does that mean that all those who claim to be able to help you lose weight or get in shape are using quackery?

No, but this section we are going to go over some of the ways that you can spot the signs of quackery in the real world.

Have you ever taken notice of just how often we are bombarded with "get fit quick" gimmicks? How often do you see a magazine cover with "lose x amount of weight in 10 days", or the "lose 5 inches off of your waist by using product xyz!" These products and statements are everywhere, you see them in commercials, on billboards, and they are in our lives everyday all day. Have you ever fallen for them? Honestly millions fall for these inflated claims all of the time, there is a reason why we see them so often, because people want to believe that they will work and they buy the products. The sad truth is that most of these products you see are just money grabs with outrageous claims. So now we are going to go over how you can spot quackery when it pertains to diets, supplements and workout equipment.

Does the products claims sound too good to be true? Is it promoting a quick fix to a problem that is complex? Like the things I mentioned above if the product is claiming that you will lose 10 pounds in 2 days or some variation of that then it is likely quackery. Health and weight loss is a long process if you see a product offering a short cut then it is likely an inflated claim. Next, does the product or advertisement play on fear? You will see this often with supplements and detox style products. These products will often play on your fear that your body is riddled with toxins and you must use their product to detox if you want to lose weight and be healthy. Often you will see a supplement claim that you won't ever get all of the nutrients your body needs from food alone and you have to take their special pill to fill in the gaps. Our bodies are amazing machines and we have made it this long without needing a special pill or detox foot massagers to keep us going. With a proper diet that covers the main food groups you will not have to worry about not getting enough nutrients, outside of any special medical problems. The same goes for detox products, our bodies have organs that remove toxins and waste products from our bodies. If you have a special medical condition that is preventing your organs from performing their detox functions then you should be consulting your doctor and not the infomercial on at 6 am.

Keep an eye out for before and after pictures. You will see this often with weight loss pills and special workout equipment. Not only can pictures be photo shopped but angles and lighting can really manipulate an image. When looking at the before and after pictures look for certain signs of quackery. In the before pictures often the person is slouching forward with their shoulders rolled and their belly pushed out. Notice their skin tone; it is usually much whiter than the after picture. This is done through excessive lighting preventing any shadows in the before picture and having more favorable lighting and possibly a tan in the second picture. Why do they do this? A darker skin tone or lighting that allows the body to cast shadows on itself will show more definition and make you look more fit/athletic. Angles can help to add a more fit look to a person as well, often a before picture is just a straight on shot while in the after picture the person might be posing while standing or twisting into an angle. Finally look at the difference in posture. In the before pictures a person usually has poor posture while in the after picture the person is standing up straight with their shoulders back and have their chest inflated to give a better look.

Don't be afraid to ask for credentials if someone is trying to sell you something in person or over the phone. We all have friends that sell those fat fighter style products and the lose weight quick wraps. The people making the claims and selling those products on their Facebook page or in front of the super market will unlikely have any credentials when it comes to the product. All they can do is parrot the claims that they were told to push. A red flag should always go up if they are using terms like "natural" or trying to speak over your head with medical jargon that is unnecessary. Often time's people will use medical jargon to hide false claims. Check into any products claims and research it thoroughly, it will almost always be too good to be true.

Finally with fitness equipment remember what we have learned so far. Not all exercises target all of your muscles! So if you see a commercial with a guy or girl that is very fit and muscular and the claim is that they got that way by using their product then it is likely quackery. A certain weight that you shake comes to mind doesn't it? When a fitness product has limited uses then you will likely get limited results from it. Simply shaking a 5 or 10 pound weight with your arm is not going to give you defined legs or glutes like the people in the commercial. It might build up some strength in that arm but not enough to make you look like the model.

So how do you know if a product is worth your time, effort, or money? Look for products that promote movement and hard work. If the product looks like it is being used to try to make an exercise easier or over complicating simple exercise then it's likely not worth your money. You can see examples of this in products that are meant to engage your abs. Look at the product carefully, does it look like you use momentum to complete the exercise or is there a focus on using your muscles? Does it take something simple like a sit-up or crunch and complicate it with unneeded chairs or other equipment? Chances are if it does then you shouldn't waste your time. Look for products that can have multiple uses, and things you can see yourself doing. One that comes to mind is something like the total gym. You can use it to work out several different areas of the body and the workout is as easy or as hard as you want it to be.

So to end this section there are thousands of get fit quick products or weight loss pills and supplements that are not worth your time or money and simply will not work. The key is to be able to spot the signs that the product is using quackery to try to trick you into buying it. If you want to try at home workout equipment, thoroughly research the product to make sure that it will actually promote what you want to get out of it. Not all products out there are false; knowing how to spot the quackery could keep you from wasting your time and becoming discouraged with your lack of results.

33

Your scale could be Fake News

Losing weight really boils down to the idea that you want a certain number to pop up on that scale when you step on it. Do you obsess over that scale? Do you step on it every day or several times a day? Do you get mad when you step on it and it hasn't changed or reads a number higher than the day before even though you have been doing everything right!? The truth is that the number on the scale is important but it is not always a great representation of your progress when viewed in the short time frame of a day or two.

Your weight can fluctuate 5 to 10 pounds in a given day for a variety of reasons, so one day you might weight 200 pounds and the next you weigh 203 pounds than later that evening you might weigh 198 pounds. The truth is that we have a base weight that is our true weight and we have a range that our weight will change either up or down and this can depend on a variety of factors. The most common factors are usually water retention, food weight, urination and bowel movements. When you eat foods that are high in carbohydrates or salt our bodies tend to retain more water, and likewise throughout the day the foods that we eat and drink have a physical weight to them that we are adding to our bodies. So weighing yourself following a meal will show an increase in weight.

How can we get an accurate weight? I am sure you have heard all sorts of different opinions on this topic, but what is the best method? The best way that I can suggest is to weigh yourself first thing every morning after you use the bathroom. To get the most consistent results you should use the same scale every time and check your weight while you're naked. A different scale could give a different number and the physical weight of your clothes can vary a great deal. Be sure that you are recording your weight every day, I recommend using an app or a spreadsheet that can collect the data and put it in a line graph. Using the graphs you can see the progress as a visual representation and can see your weight go down.

As you lose weight you will see that your weight although might be fluctuating it is still declining overtime. Monitoring and recording your weight allows you to keep a close eye on how you are doing with your diet and exercise. If you are noticing that your weight loss is slowing down over the period of several days or weeks then you will need to make adjustments to your calorie intake and exercise. This is an important part of the process to keeping you on track to reach your goals!

34

Muscles of the Body: Chest

Turing in a different direction I want to use some of the sections of this book to cover the various muscle groups of the body. I feel that having an understanding about what muscles are in each region of the body and what function they perform is important. This is because as you go forward through this journey you will come across information and topics that require you to have an understanding about your muscles. Knowing what functions your muscles perform is a great way for you to form a mind muscle connection during exercise. The mind muscle connection will be an important subject covered later in this book.

Looking at the anatomy of the chest we are going to consider 3 muscles. The Pectoralis Major, Pectoralis Minor, and the Serratus Anterior. When discussing what the muscles of the chest do, you will probably hear this group called the pusher muscles. The reason why is due to what movements they are tasked with performing. Let's take a closer look at what each of the 3 muscles do! The Pectorals major is the biggest muscle of the chest, I am sure the major gave that away though. It is a large fan shaped muscle that originates in your clavicle (collar bone) ribs and sternum (center of your chest). It connects to the upper part of your humerus, which is the bone of your upper arm between your elbow and shoulder joints. One of the main functions of the pectoralis major is to move your arms across your chest. This is why it is considered a pusher muscle, because the action of moving your arms across your chest will cause your arms to push out in front of your body.

The Pectoralis Minor is smaller than the major and is located underneath the larger pectoralis major. It is a thin triangle shaped muscle that originates at 3rd, 4th, and 5th ribs and attaches to your scapula (shoulder blade). Its main function is to help pull the shoulder blade forward and down. I have added the Serratus anterior to the chest muscles due to its close proximity to the other 2 and it has similar function to the pectoralis minor. The serratus anterior is a small muscle that connects the ribs to the shoulder blades. It is tasked with pulling the shoulder blades forward and upward. Of the 3 muscles mentioned the pectoralis major is the easiest to visually see on the body as it is the largest, the minor is located under the major and is not visible. The serratus anterior can be visible but might lack in muscle definition and size to be noticeable, although if you can see it you will notice that it has an appearance like that of a serrated knife.

Now that we know what the muscles of the chest are and what purpose they serve, what are ways we can exercise them? Knowing that they are considered pushers we know that any pushing exercise will work them out. These can include things like bench press, push-ups, chest fly's, incline bench press, decline bench press and so on. Basically any movement that involves pushing a weight away from the body, or bringing a weight from the side of the body to the front through the movement of the humerus will exercise the muscles of the chest. Knowing what actions your muscle groups perform will allow you to specifically target them in exercise to increase their strength, endurance, size, and appearance. The next time you perform any exercise that involves pushing, such as doing a push-up, focus on the chest muscle as you go. You will begin to pick out and feel the muscle groups contract and work, building the mind muscle connection.

35

How to Understand Nutritional labels

You have been working really hard on making better food choices controlling your portions and adding exercise into you daily lives. We briefly covered reading a part of a nutritional label very early on in this book, now we are going to take a more in-depth look at how to read a nutritional label and what specifics you should be looking for.

Something that you may or may not notice when looking at nutritional labels is that they are all standard. Each label has 6 basic sections for specific information, 5 of which are divided by a thick black line. The sections start at the top of the label and go down. Section 1 contains the serving size; section 2 shows the total calories and calories from fat per serving. We have already covered this section earlier so we will not spend time on it again. Sections 3 and 4 show the nutrients in the food, and how much of each.

The nutrients in section 3 are the ones that you should try to limit, these include the fat, saturated fat, Trans fat, cholesterol, and sodium. Having some of these is alright and somewhat unavoidable; however you should try to limit them as much as you can. Section 4 shows the nutrients that you should try to get more of. These are your fibers, vitamins and minerals including calcium and iron. The 5th section is known as the footnotes, and shows the standard percent daily value that is recommended based on a 2,000 calorie a day diet. Depending on the size of the label this may or may not be on the label, it is also the same on every label when it is present.

The 6th and final section is "Percent Daily Value"; it can be abbreviated as %DV and is located on the right side of the label. This section tells you what percentage of your daily need is in the food based on a 2,000 calorie a day diet. For example the label might say this food item has 20% you daily value of calcium for the day. So you know that you need to get another 80% of your daily value for calcium for the day from another source. It is a good rule of thumb that if the daily value shows 5% or lower then it is a low amount, and a daily percent of 20% is high.

So take a moment after this section and look at a few of your favorite foods labels in your cabinets. Do you see high percentages in the 3rd sections? What about the 4th sections? Are the serving sizes big or small? Do you see high calorie content with low serving sizes? The key is to have a balanced diet in your life, cutting out whole food groups is not always the way to go. Understanding that you can have foods that are not always that great for you but being mindful of you Percent Daily Value could set you up for long term sustainable success!

So how can you use this to your advantage? Can you set yourself up for success with the foods you purchase? Think on this for a moment, what actions can you take? The truth is we live in the greatest point in human history as it pertains to the food availability. We can go to the supermarket and see 5 different options for the same food products. The food products might appear to be the same in appearance, price, and taste but are they identical? The answer is no, they can vary a great deal in calories, portion size, and nutrition. Knowing this and understanding nutritional labels means that you can decide to stock your kitchen with good choices before ever leaving the store. On your next grocery trip try comparing nutritional labels between the products you usually buy and the other similar products available. You might be able to replace your current choices with similar products that have fewer calories and better nutrition! Keep in mind that these differences might not be huge but if you have learned anything so far it's that the small things can really add up to big things in a short period of time. Setting yourself up for long term success starts with the choices you make, and for your nutritional choices that means making the correct choices in the grocery aisles!

36

Calories Continued

From section 1 in this book you can see that I am a proponent of calories in vs calories out. In fact I made the statement a calorie is a calorie is a calorie. I also mentioned that there can be a big difference in the nutrition that is included in a calorie. In the last section we touched a little on the differences in nutrition within our foods so in this section we are going to expand a little on that concept. You might be thinking to yourself that if a calorie is a calorie than why should I worry about nutrition when the goal is to lose weight? The answer to that is pretty simple, just losing weight won't mean you are healthy if you develop malnutrition.

Malnutrition is the state of having a lack of proper nutrition. This was common back in the old days due to a lack of food; however it is becoming a growing problem in today's society as well. The reason for this can be found in the food labels you were looking at in the last section. Some foods you eat could be low in essential nutrients that our bodies need to sustain ourselves, and if we are regularly eating those types of foods it is easy to have nutritional deficiency in certain nutrients. So as you can see it is possible to be overweight or obese and be malnourished, it all depends on what you are eating. You could be consuming high calorie low nutritional foods! What are some of the symptoms of malnutrition you might be wondering? You could develop weak muscles, a feeling of being low, and a general tired feeling all of the time. Another major effect can be a reduction in your ability to fight of illness and infection. Do any of those apply to you?

Remember a calorie is just a unit of energy to our bodies, but our bodies need far more than just energy to run. They need a wide variety of nutrients to keep operating at peak performance. What are these nutrients though? Well there are 7 basic categories to nutrients that we are going to cover more in depth in the following sections. You might have noticed the 7 categories on the nutrition labels already. They are as follows Carbohydrates, fats, fiber, minerals, proteins, vitamins, and water. These nutrients can be divided into 2 different groups, Macronutrients and Micronutrients, commonly referred to as macro and micros. The macros include carbohydrates, fats, fiber, water and protein. These are the nutrients you require more of in your diets. The micros include your vitamins and minerals; you need these in a smaller quantity.

All of the nutrients we consume play an important role within our bodies. Some build muscles, while others keep our bones strong. Some provide energy while others maintain nerve health. The key is to make sure that you are eating a balanced diet rich in nutrients! This will keep you feeling better in mind, body, and spirit!

37

Nutrients: Carbohydrates

In the last section we very briefly discussed that there is more to your health than just counting calories. Yes calories in vs calories out are the keys to losing weight but this book is about your health. Losing weight is great for your health but being malnourished is not. We are now going to look at each of those 7 basics categories of nutrients, starting with carbohydrates.

Are all carbs created equally? No. The category of carbs can be broken down into 3 other group's monosaccharides, disaccharides, and polysaccharides. Those are some big words with fairly simple meanings so let's break the terms down so we are on the same page. As you read those words you will have noticed that the root of the 3 words were the same, saccharide. This term is just another name for sugar! Now let's look at the prefix of each term. Mono meaning one, di meaning 2, and finally poly meaning many (3+). So we can look at it likes this, Monosaccharides means 1 sugar, disaccharides means 2 sugars, and polysaccharides meaning 3 or more sugars. It is important to note that this is on a carbs molecular level in order to understand the following information.

We have all heard that there are good carbs and bad carbs or simple carbs and complex carbs, but is that true? For the most part you can think of it as that way. As I mentioned this is looking at carbohydrates on a molecular level. So what makes a carb simple or complex? Well the amount of sugars. A good carb is more complex so this is the polysaccharides, while the simple or "bad" carbs are the mono and disaccharides. This is where it becomes complex on a molecular level. When you have a monosaccharide you have a single sugar molecular, which means your body doesn't need to do anything to beak the sugar down. It can just be absorbed very quickly, and this can lead to both spikes in blood sugar and quick digestion. If food is too quickly digested then hunger feelings can return quickly and if weight loss is the goal you can see how this can make things harder on yourself.

When there is more than one sugar in the carb then the body has to break them down because the sugars are chemically bonded together. Think back to your old chemistry lessons, to break down bonds energy needs to be used. For disaccharides we are talking about 2 sugars that are bonded together, so the body will have to use a little energy to break the bond. This means that it will take a little longer to digest as well as burning a little energy to accomplish it. Taking longer to digest means that your blood sugar levels will remain more constant and you will feel fuller longer. Finally looking at the polysaccharides, following the same principle of breaking chemical bonds you can see how these are the "good carbs". This is because the poly carbs will take the longest to break down and burn the most energy in the process. So you are burning energy to make energy making weight loss easier, and helping to maintain a feeling of being full longer. With the added benefit of keeping a stable blood sugar level, as we learned earlier can help to prevent disease and illness.

Now we have an understanding of what carbohydrates are on a chemical and molecular level, but what are they when it comes to foods? You can find them as part of foods like rice, noodles, breads and any grain based product. Perfect, now we know what foods have carbs in them! Wait, but how do we tell which foods have good or bad carbs in them?

There are somethings that you can look for that will give a clue as to which carbs are in your foods.

If the food you are eating is not refined then there is a good chance that it will contain more complex carbs. This is commonly referred to as "whole foods" and can include your vegetables, fruit, potatoes, and whole grains. A good indicator can be the darkness of the product as well. For example, whole grain bread is typically a darker brown, whereas refined grains will give a lighter color such as in white breads and white flours. If the food you are eating is more refined or has added sugars then you are likely consuming simple carbs. This can include sweetened beverages, fruit juices, white breads, pastas, and white rice.

You might be wondering how much of our diet should carbs make up? Carbohydrates are big contributor to the energy our bodies need, because of this it is recommended that carbs make up 45-65 percent of your daily calories. So at 2,000 calorie a day that would mean you should be eating between 900 and 1,300 calories from carbs a day. This translates to between 225 and 325 grams of carbs a day. Hold up, I thought we were talking about calories from carbs, why did you bring grams into this!? On a nutritional label carbs are measured in grams, and there are 4 grams per calorie of carbohydrate. This means figuring out how many grams of carbs you need/eat requires an extra step of math.

At this point you know how to read a nutritional label and now you have a very good understanding of what a carbohydrate is. As is common with sections in this book it is time to apply what you have learned. You know your TDEE, so you know how many calories you should be eating a day to maintain your current weight, and you are currently running in a calorie deficit that is about 15 to 25 percent below your TDEE. It is time to take the actual number of calories you eat and check if you are consuming the correct amount of carbs. So take your current calorie intake and multiply to find the range between 45 and 65 percent. You then take those two numbers within that range and divide each of them by 4, because 4 grams of carbs make up 1 calorie. This will give you a range for carbs in grams. Now you simply count your grams of carbs during the day and see if you are above or below that range. The important thing is to find what works best for you. Some people can be fine well below that range while others are not. Keeping a low carb diet can make it easier to maintain a low calorie diet in many cases!

38

Nutrients: Fats

The last section was very complicated when it came to understanding carbohydrates; I hope that you find this section on fats to be just as informative and maybe a little less complex. As the title shows we will be covering fats from a nutritional and dietary stand point. As you will learn this is very different from the information that we previously covered on body fat. Nutrient fats can be broken down into 3 subgroups known as saturated fats, unsaturated fats, and Tran's fats.

Saturated fats are fats that will appear solid at room temperature; this can include things like butters, dairy products and lards. The fat that is found in animal meets such as beef, pork and chicken belong to the saturated fat category. The American Heart Association recommends that your diet only has 5-6 percent of your daily calories be from saturated fats. This is because saturated fats have been linked to raising the level of cholesterol in your blood. High levels of LDL cholesterol can increase your risk of heart disease and stroke. For the women reading this book keep in mind that heart disease is the number one killer of women, so why increase your risk by eating too many saturated fats?

Unsaturated fats are typically liquid at room temperature. These can include the fats that are found in fish such as salmon, trout, tuna, and herring. They are also found in your plant based foods such as avocados, olives and nuts like almonds and walnuts. Several of your cooking oils will fall into this category as well, including vegetable oils and olive oils. Unlike saturated fats unsaturated fats may help to improve your bad cholesterol when they replace unsaturated fats in your diet.

You may see unsaturated fats represented as Monounsaturated on a nutritional label, which is generally found in almonds, hazelnuts, pecans, olive, canola, and peanut oils. You might also see these fats referred to as polyunsaturated fats on the nutritional label. You can find polyunsaturated fats in sunflower, corn, soybean, and flaxseed oils, as well as fish and walnuts.

The final type of fat we are covering is the Tran's fats. This type of fat is found in small amounts in dairy and meats but it is mostly man made. It is created through a process that adds hydrogen to vegetable oil. This causes the oil to become more of a solid when stored at room temperatures. Tran's fats are used to increase a foods shelf life because the hydrogenated oil is less likely to spoil. You can commonly find these in baked goods like cakes, and cookies as well as fried snacks like chips. Tran's fats are seen as the worst type of fat because it is known to raise your bad cholesterol (LDL) and lower your good cholesterol (HDL). This can lead to heart disease.

It is recommended that your daily percent of calories from fat should fall between 20-35 percent. Figuring out how many you need we can follow the same basic math from the carbohydrate section, with a few changes in the numbers. So first take how many calories you are currently eating daily and find how many calories are in the range from 20-35 percent. For a 2000 calorie a day diet this would be between 400 and 700 calories. As you can tell on a nutritional label fats are shown the same way as carbohydrates, in grams. So to find out how many grams of fat are in that range we need to do the same thing we did with the carbohydrates. We need to divide the calories in our range by the number of grams of fat in a single calorie. There is a big difference here though! Unlike carbs which have 4 grams per calorie, fats have 9 grams per calorie. So we will need to divide by 9. For our example this means that in a 2,000 calorie a day diet you should eat between 44 to 78 grams of fat, and the majority of those grams should come from unsaturated fats!

It is now time to apply this new found information to your day to day life. Just like the carbohydrate section you should keep track of your fat intake by counting the grams of fat you eat based on the information provided on the nutritional label. Are you getting enough fats? Are they the good types of unsaturated fats, or are you consuming more of the saturated and Tran's fats? Remember you do not have to cut out all of the fats in your diet, you should just be mindful of what kinds of fats you are consuming and if you are over representing fats in your daily diet.

39

Nutrients: Fiber

We hear all the time from doctors and commercials about the benefits of fiber. How it helps with digestion and makes you regular. How it can reduce your risk of disease as well as other digestive issues. All of that is true but what is lacking is information on what fiber actually is and why it helps with those things! This section we will briefly go over a little information on what fiber is and how it can benefit us.

Fiber is the indigestible parts of plant based foods. It is actually a type of carbohydrate, but what makes it different from other carbohydrates is that the body can't digest it. If you recall back to the section about carbohydrates we know that carbs are broken down into sugar molecules, since fiber cannot be digested it does not get broken down into sugars. In fact it passes through the body undigested. What is the point then, you may be asking. Fiber can actually help regulate the body's use of sugars by slowing down digestion and allowing for blood sugar to remain steadier. It can also aid in weight loss by making you feel fuller longer.

There are two types of fiber, soluble and insoluble. Soluble fibers can be dissolved in water, and during the digestive process it becomes a gel like substance. This gel helps to slow down the digestive process. You can find soluble fiber in several foods including oatmeal, nuts, beans, apples, and lentils. On the other side we have insoluble fibers. This type of fiber typically retains its shape as it passes through our body. However this fiber helps to speed up digestion, which can keep you regular and prevent constipation. You can find insoluble fiber in whole wheat, whole grain, brown rice, legumes, cucumbers and carrots. The best sources for both types of fiber include whole grain foods, fresh fruits and vegetables, legumes, and nuts. Basically any plant based food source.

Now you know what fiber is and where it comes from, you also know that it can affect our digestive system. Now what are the benefits of introducing it into our diets? A study done by Harvard found that a diet high in fiber showed a linked to a lower risk of heart disease by 40%. We have already reviewed type 2 diabetes so we know the risks associated with high blood sugar. We now know that fiber can help to regulate blood sugar, it should not come as a surprise to you that diets low in fiber and high in foods that cause quick increases in blood sugar levels, more than doubles your risk of type 2 diabetes. Finally as mentioned several times now that fiber helps to keep us regular. Constipation is the most common gastrointestinal complaint in America. Increasing your fiber intake can both relieve as well as prevent constipation.

Much like many of the nutrients we have learned about, Americans typically do not get enough fiber in their daily diets. It is recommended that you get between 22 and 34 grams of fiber every day. The average American only consumes about 15 grams a day, which is not far off the minimum recommendation. Looking at that stat you can see that only a slight increase in fiber intake for the average American could greatly increase their quality of life!

The same as the other nutrient sections track your daily fiber intake to see if you are meeting the 22 to 34 grams a day. However if you are finding that your fiber intake is low do not try to increase it too quickly. Increasing your fiber intake to quickly can cause digestive discomfort and other issues, you will need to increase your fiber intake slowly over a couple of weeks to give your body the time it needs to adjust. It is recommended that as you increase your fiber you increase your water consumption as well.

40

Nutrients: Protein

It is time to tackle the nutrient protein, which might be more complicated than you first thought. As we all know protein is the building block of life, it is found in our muscles, bone, hair, skin, basically all body parts and tissues. It is in our blood and makes up enzymes that perform chemical reactions. As you can tell protein is very important! So we should focus on getting protein no matter the source, right? Not really, quality of protein source matters just as much as quantity!

To start we need to understand where protein comes from. Of course we all know that it is in animal products like meat, chicken, and fish. However you can also find protein in other sources including fruits, vegetables, grains, nuts, and seeds. Sounds like protein is in basically everything we eat, but is all protein created equally? The simple answer to that question is no. Proteins contain amino acids that our bodies use. There are a few different ways for our bodies to get these acids, first we make them ourselves or we modify others. There are a few types of amino acids that we cannot produce ourselves and they must come from the foods we eat. These amino acids are known as essential. Protein from animal sources is known as complete protein, this is because it contains all of the essential amino acids that we use. Plant based proteins are known as incomplete proteins. As you probably guessed this is because plant based proteins lack in 1 or more essential amino acid.

Since animal based protein is complete and plant based is incomplete then we should focus mostly on animal proteins, right? As I am sure you already know the answer to this question is no. There are pro's and con's to each type of protein and finding a healthy balance between the two is what we should all strive for. Due to plant based proteins being incomplete proteins you need to ensure that you are consuming a wide variety of protein sources to ensure you are getting all of the essential amino acids. On the other side animal based protein might be complete and have all of the essential amino acids but red meats can be high in saturated fats. As we have learned these are the fats you should limit. Following the same thought, ham provides a protein rich source but it is high in sodium. In fact a 6 oz. ham steak will provide 500 milligrams over your daily sodium recommendations. While plant based foods like cooked lentils can provide 18 grams of protein as well as 15 grams of fiber without saturated fats or sodium.

Seems like a mixed bag doesn't it? One source of protein could be complete but also contain unhealthy nutrients while the other might provide more healthy nutrients but might be incomplete. This is where it can be very important to monitor the nutritional labels of the foods you eat to ensure that you are meeting your dietary needs and setting yourself up for a healthy diet to meet all of your nutritional needs.

What is the daily recommendation of protein for you? Some recommend that your daily calorie intake is 10 to 35 percent protein. You can follow the same math formula that we used for carbohydrates to figure out how many grams of protein per day you should be eating. Like carbs, 1 calorie of protein is 4 grams. However there is another way to determine how much protein you should be consuming a day. You need 8 grams of protein a day per 20 pounds of body weight. Some studies show that diets high in protein and low in carbs can help with weight loss in the short term. However it is not clear if this is due to different levels of water retention between the diet subjects. Long term shows little difference between low carb high protein and balanced diets.

41

Nutrients: Minerals

I am not going to spend a great deal of time on minerals because it is likely that you are receiving enough minerals in your daily diets. This is more likely now that you have been monitoring your food intake and adding in healthier whole food choices. If you are having problems with minerals then consulting your doctor would be your best course of action. They could recommend specific dietary advice or supplements that would aid you.

Although I do not wish to spend a great deal of time on minerals do not take that as meaning they are not important to your wellbeing. The truth is without the minerals we get in our diets many of our body systems and functions would suffer. For example you need iron to make hemoglobin, the part of your blood that attaches to oxygen. Calcium builds bones and teeth as well as being essential for nerves to send messages. Without calcium our nerves couldn't tell our muscles to move! Potassium helps to balance your fluids and maintain your heart beat. Zinc aids in blood clots and improves our immune systems. There are many others and if I spent time going over each of them this section would be very long!

I have mentioned it in several other sections, having a balanced diet where you are getting your recommended amounts of each food group will make it possible to be getting your daily value of nutrients. For minerals this is no different. If you are including a variety of vegetables, fruits, whole grains, beans, protein, and dairy products then you will likely not have to worry about your mineral intake. It is important to mention that we cannot manufacture the minerals in our own bodies; we must get them from our diets. So where do they come from? They are found in the soil, rocks, and water from the earth, and absorbed by the plants. This is why you can find minerals in fresh plant based foods, but it also explains why we can get minerals from animal based foods. Animals eat the plants and absorb the minerals just like us, and if we eat the animal we absorb those minerals second hand.

It is also common to find processed foods that have been fortified or enriched with minerals. You can see this commonly in breakfast cereals, as well as different supplements pills and powders. I hope this section was able to drive the idea about the benefits of a balanced diet home for you. Unlike the other sections I am not going to go over the recommended daily amount due to their being so many different minerals that we need. If you are concerned that you are not getting enough minerals in your diets please consult your doctor.

42

Nutrients: Vitamins

Much like the previous section on minerals I do not wish to spend a great deal of time on vitamins. This, like the minerals, is because there are too many to go through that it would make this section insufferably long, and that you are likely getting enough vitamins in your daily diets. However there are some things that you should understand when we are talking about vitamins!

Much like minerals vitamins play a big role in maintaining our body and systems. Thiamin (Vitamin B1) is needed for healthy muscles, hair as well as brain and nerve function. Ascorbic acid (vitamin c) could lower your risk of cancers, and bolster the immune system. Calciferol (vitamin D) can maintain normal blood levels of calcium and can be absorbed through the skin from the Sun. Folic Acid can help with new cell creation and may reduce the risk of heart disease. All of these things sound great so should you be taking a multi vitamin to ensure you are getting enough vitamins and bridge the any gaps left by your diet?

I am not going to recommend taking or not taking a vitamin supplement. Decisions such as that should be discussed with your doctor. Having too much of a vitamin can be a bad thing. For example to much vitamin C could cause stomach cramps or nausea. Although it is rare having too much vitamin D could result in a buildup of calcium in your blood which could cause weakness and vomiting. Like all things we discuss in these pages moderation is important.

The last part of this section will be covering where to find vitamins in your diet. You might be noticing the trend here and know what I am going to tell you before you even read it. Eating a diet rich in fresh fruits and vegetables as well as whole grains healthy oils and nuts will provide you with all or most of the vitamins you need. Doing this should prevent any deficiencies, but if you are worried that your diet change or current diet is not going to provide you with enough, consult your doctor.

43

Nutrients: Water and the importance of staying hydrated

I know that we have been on a long stretch of talking about nutrients and I am sure you have been getting tired of the same topic being discussed for a week straight. Trust me I was getting bored writing it. That being said the information was very important for you to fully understand nutritional labels and good diet choices going forward. Today we will be briefly going over the importance of water and staying hydrated. After this section we will be done with nutrition for a little while.

Make sure you get your 8 glasses of water in everyday! That's a phrase we hear often that is easier said than done. I know people who could drink 8 glasses of water by lunch and I know people who struggle to drink 3 all day. Have you ever tried to drink 8 glasses of water in a day? It is not fun for most people. Well you might be relieved to know that the "drink 8 glasses a day" was more of a guideline and not based in actual science!

So if the recommendation is not 8 glasses a day then what is it? Truth is I can't tell you; in fact it really depends on to many individual factors to have a concrete amount recommendation. Not overly helpful, right? Well let's go over some of those factors and then I can give you a recommendation on what you can aim for. Individual water needs can change based on a person's size, age, activity level, time of the year and so on. Studies also show that obese people tend to be more dehydrated than people of a healthy weight. It is also not a surprise that if you are more active you will need to consume more water to replace water lost during and after activity, and that during hotter times of the year you will naturally sweat more.

Staying hydrated has many benefits for both health and weight loss strategies. First up are some obvious health benefits. Staying hydrated can affect your bodies waste removal processes. Yes it helps you to use the bathroom more effectively and makes it easier on your kidneys to remove nitrogen from your blood. Your kidneys use water to remove waste products creating urine. When you are dehydrated your kidneys will try to retain water for use in other parts of the body. This causes your urine to become darker in color and have more of an odor. On the other end (no pun intended) when you are dehydrated your colon will remove water from your stool which can lead to constipation. Remember back in our fiber section we learned that water plumps up fiber in your digestive track and that acts like a broom as it works its way out of your body.

For weight loss drinking plenty of water can help to make you feel full during the day, which helps to control hunger urges. Replacing a sugary drink with a glass of water will help to reduce your calorie intake. Finally a strategy that has shown a great deal of success is to drink more water during your meals. Doing this will cause you to feel more full and eat less food, which in turn means you are consuming fewer calories.

"So if water helps with weight loss and body maintenance, how do I know if I am getting enough?" You can find context clues more or less within your body's functions; the easiest one is in your urinations. Your urine should be light in color, or almost clear, as well as odorless. This will tell you that your body has enough water so it is able to release plenty during the production of urine in the kidneys. Easy enough? Well it is easy to have a light color in your urine following a large amount of hydration only for your urine to darken and develop an odor throughout the day. Our bodies can only hold so much water at any given time so hydrating once a day will not be enough; it is a practice you need to do regularly. You should aim to have 5-7 urinations a day that are light in color an odorless. If you are having more than this than you might be over hydrating and if you have less than this you might be under hydrating.

Remember that many factors influence how much water you need. So what was enough for one day might be too much or too little for another day. It might take some trial and error to find a balance in your life, and eventually you will find an amount of water consumption that works well for you! Just make it part of your daily commitment to remain hydrated! Much like in the other sections, do not take this as medical advice, if you are having concerns with your hydration please consult your doctor. Thirst, urination, and hydration issues can be symptoms of other medical problems such as diabetes and hypoglycemia.

44

Is this going to be forever?

One of the complaints (or reasons if you will) I
hear from people that don't want to lose weight or are having a
hard time with a restrictive diet is. "I don't want to go without X
all my life" or "I don't want to be counting calories and running
on a treadmill my whole life, I would rather just stay fat." I get
it, we are about a month and a half into this journey, I hope that
you have been slowly implementing some of the knowledge and
strategies into your life to make this a life style change and not
just another crash diet of lose and gain. Change is hard, but
once those changes are a habit is it really that hard?

I have championed this process as being a life style
change from the very beginning and I explained to you my
thoughts on why people who simply use restrictive diets gain
the weight back in 5 years. So basically to answer the question
in the title of this section, yes this is going to be forever! But,
and this is a big but, certain actions that you are taking right
now will become second nature habits. On top of that running
at a calorie deficit is not permanent; once you reach your goal
you can easily reassess your TDEE and find how many calories
you need to consume to maintain your weight loss. Sounds a lot
like I am telling you that you will be counting calories for the
rest of your life, isn't it? If you are currently struggling with this
concept well I hope I can relieve some stress about the idea in
this section.

The truth is that I am trying to ease you into a life
style of putting your health and wellbeing first, and doing so by
making healthy decisions. At this point in time you are in a
knock out drag out fight with your old habits fighting to remain

your habits and your new habits fighting to become your daily habits. Which side is winning? At this point some of your old habits are probably winning from time to time as are some of the new ones. Remember I mentioned before that new habits can take 60 days or longer to become actual habits. We are only on day 44 so if you are struggling keep going, you can win this fight! Now why am I talking about habits so much? Recall that I mentioned that counting calories would more than likely start causing you to eat healthier foods? Has that started to happen for you yet? The healthier foods typically offer more volume and nutrition while having fewer calories than the not so healthy foods. So in reality your counting calories is causing you to develop healthy eating habits!

What this means is that although your life style change towards healthier choices is intended to be forever that doesn't mean that you will have to be counting calories for the rest of your life. Think about it for a moment here, before picking up this book and deciding to make a change what was your diet like? You probably consumed the same types of foods regularly, correct? Sure you might have changed it up from time to time but you likely stuck with the same old same old, and on top of that portion control was probably never a thought. Now where are you, are you replacing your old normal diet with a new normal? By this I mean has some of the healthier foods and meals that you have been eating started to become your new regular meals? Has portion control started to become a habit? Are you beginning to naturally put less food on your plate? Are you starting to think to yourself "well I shouldn't eat much of this, but I can have more of that"?

The point is that as you make these new habits your permanent habits you will no longer need to watch your calories so closely. You will naturally eat the healthier choices just like you use to naturally eat the unhealthy choices. You will naturally fill your plate with the appropriate amount just like you use to naturally over eat. Your body will adjust to be happy with the portions you are eating. This is called your maintenance mode, where you just maintain your body weight by maintaining your healthy habits. Once you reach your maintenance mode you will be able to make small adjustments from time to time based on your weight. For example you might step on the scale and see you gained 8 pounds or notice that your pants are getting a little tighter. Then you make a slight adjustment to how you are eating and lose those extra pounds before the weight becomes a problem again. It will be a whole lot easier to just maintain your habits to maintain your weight and if you slip up a little early intervention will make it so you can quickly and easily return back to your goal weight.

So you can see that setting up healthy habits will do the work of maintaining your weight loss for you. Yes from time to time you might need to monitor your calorie intake if you start to gain back some weight, but you have the tools to make small changes when that time comes to return to your goal weight. The point is that at this moment you might be having a hard time with staying motivated to keep up these changes. Know that one day these changes in your habits will happen without thought, and one day all of this will become easy. Putting in the work now will pay off big in the near future.

45

Exercise: Lunge

Moving along with our exercise sections we are going to go over a very simple but effective body weight exercise. The lunge is a lower body exercise that can really activate all of the major muscle groups of your legs as well as your core. The main movers will be your quads (the muscles on the front of your legs) your hamstrings (the muscles on the back of your legs) and your glutes (your butt). It is great for building both muscle strength and endurance.

The lunge is similar to a squat except you focus on one leg at a time. For this reason it is a great beginner exercise because it prevents building a muscle imbalance. A muscle imbalance happens when someone does an exercise and focuses more on one side than the other. This can cause the muscles to strengthen and grow differently, and is something you should avoid doing.

To perform the lunge you start from a standing position with your feet about hip width apart. You will next take a big step forward with your right leg. Shift your weight forward so that your right heel makes contact with the ground. Begin to lower your body towards the ground so that your left knee bends and lowers towards the ground. Stop when your right thigh is parallel to the ground and your left thigh is vertical. You can stop lowering to the ground once your left knee is almost to the ground, as you become more familiar with the exercise you can lightly tap your left knee against the ground. It is important to not let your right knee extend out past your toes, so you do not want too much of a forward lean. From this position press the right heel into the ground to press yourself back up to your starting standing position. Repeat by stepping forward with your left leg and lowering your right knee to the ground.

This can be a difficult exercise depending on your fitness level. You might find that you are only able to do a couple for each side before you fatigue. Like all of the other exercises just keep working at it and you will slowly improve. Try adding it to your daily routine by doing a few minutes of lunges a day!

46

Sitting 8 hours a Day is as Bad as Smoking

We live in a society that has allowed for our occupations to require more sitting and less physical labor. Not everyone has the luxury or curse of an office type job where you sit most of the day however since the 1960's jobs in the US that require at least moderate physical activity have gone from 50 percent down to 20 percent of occupations. This means that 80 percent of current jobs in the country require only light or no physical activity. So there is a good chance that the people reading this book have a job where you sit for a good portion of the day if not the entire day. This habit of sitting all day though can be harder on your body than you ever imagined.

I have some firsthand anecdotal experience in this. I was a decathlete in college and an athlete all throughout high school. After college I worked for several years in a food distribution warehouse. This job had me on my feet for walking and picking up boxes for 8 or more hours a day. On a busy day my Fitbit would tell me I walked around 28 thousand steps. Then I got a different job, one where I spend all day at my desk on my computer. I very much enjoy my job, however I can tell a difference in how I feel now that I am not as active. I have made it a priority to get up and move every hour as well as getting in at least an hour of physical activity a day. Without doing this I feel that 2 o'clock lull where I am tired and looking for some caffeine, but that is only a temporary fix and I would return back to a tired state for the rest of the day. Adding in activity during the day completely reversed this feeling and helped me to have more energy and a better mood all day and night.

Now you have heard my personal story let's look at what the research tells us. To put it bluntly sitting for 8 hours a day coupled with a sedentary life style could increase your risk of premature death by 60 percent. This means that sitting all day and not being active is as great of a risk to your health as being a smoker. Just think what you might be doing to your body if you do both. But how does sitting all day actually hurt us? There are many adverse effects and we are going to go over several of them in the following pages.

Did you know that the muscles of your legs help your heart pump your blood? It's true the muscles of your legs help return your blood to your heart against the influence of gravity that wants to cause your blood to pool in your legs. This is the process called skeletal muscle pump. Sitting can cause your heart to have to work harder to return the blood back to the heart. On top of that research has shown that sitting for long periods of time can result in your muscles burning less fat which in turn makes it easier for fatty acids to build up and clog your heart. This can greatly increase your risk of heart disease. This slow in blood flow will also decrease your brain functions as your brain does not get fresh oxygenated blood.

Posture problems can develop from prolonged sitting. It is very easy for us to forget about our posture as we sit hunched over our key boards all day. You might begin to strain your neck and shoulders because you are probably holding you head and neck out from your body or when you're on your computer or when you are on the phone. Not only might your muscles become sore and strained you might damage your vertebrae, which could lead to permanent issues and pain. As you might imagine neck problems could lead to back problems as well. Sitting for extended periods of time can reduce the flexibility of your spine and disks leading to more pain and discomfort. When sitting all day it is important to make a conscious effort to keep your shoulders back, your neck straight, and you back straight. Failing to do so might have consequences for other organs as well. Hunching over like we tend to do at a desk compresses your organs, most notably your digestive system. Compressing your digestive organs can greatly slow down the process of digestion. This can lead to bloating, cramping, constipation and heart burn. It has also been associated with dysbiosis in your gastrointestinal track. A condition that is caused by microbial imbalances in your body.

The research shows that sitting for extended periods of time can take years off your life. The *British Journal of Sports Medicine* found that for people after the age of 25 could reduce their life expectancy by 22 minutes per hour of TV watched. To put that into perspective it is reported that smoking a cigarette could reduce your life span by 11 minutes per cigarette. Other research shows that adults who spend 6 hours a day sitting and watching TV will have a reduction in life expectancy by about 5 years.

Although you are seeing a lot of research saying that you could lose 22 minutes per hour of TV or 5 years if you watch an average of 6 hours of TV a day the point that they can all agree on is that sitting for extended periods of time will reduce your life expectancy. Have you begun being more proactive about increasing your movements? We have reviewed NEAT and how adding movements and exercise can help you to lose weight and maybe alleviate aches and pains. Now you know that being sedentary might just be slowly killing you. If you haven't taken my advice to move more maybe this section was enough to convince you. But what can you do to move more throughout the day?

47

Increasing your activity: At work

The last section might have gotten you a little down, talking about disease and other ailments that can develop as a result of something you might not really be able to control. We all have to work and many of us work jobs that don't allow a lot of movement. It can be difficult to prevent some of the things mentioned in the last section like being bent over a computer all day when your job requires you to be typing all day. So I presented a problem that many of us face and now we are going to go over some solutions in the next few sections. We have already gone over a few ideas on how to increase your movements at work but we are going to take the time to expand on this a little more.

Let's start with the obvious, walk when you can! If you are able to walk to work then walk to work as often as you can. Some of you might be fortunate enough to live close to your job, maybe it is a couple blocks away or less than a mile. Some of you might not have that luxury, in fact 1 in 10 of you rely on public transportation to get to work. If you find yourself in this category then you could get off the bus a stop or two early and walk the remainder of the way to your destination. This is an easy way to add in extra activity to your day! If you drive to work park at the far end of the parking lot, remember it is about 5 steps per parking spot so you could be adding hundreds of extra steps a day or week just by parking further away. Take the stairs instead of the elevator, or if that is too many stairs at this point in time get off the elevator 1 floor early. Once that becomes easier make it 2 floors early then 3 and so on. Organize a walking group, there are usually people in your office that would be willing to walk on breaks and join your fitness journey.

"All of that sounds great but I still have to sit at my desk for the majority of the day!" That is true, you are at work to work so it is not like you can just leave your desk to go workout. So bring the workout to your desk! There are several ways that you can do this, from equipment made for your desk to special chairs and standing desks. We have all seen those stability ball chairs that you replace your desk chair with. The idea is that the sitting on the stability ball makes your seat unstable, so you will be constantly tighten your core, back and leg muscles to keep yourself balanced. This might be an option for you, however if you are like me and you are not willing to trade in your office chair for a giant bouncy ball then a stability cushion might be the way to go. These cushions are a cheaper alternative to the stability ball chairs while offering similar results. The cushion is similar to a mostly deflated beach ball that you place on your seat. The cushion makes your seat a little more unstable and forces you to tighten your core muscle up to keep yourself balanced; it could also improve your desk posture as well. It might not work as well as sitting on a full sized stability ball but it could give similar results for a much lower price.

Beyond just having a chair that forces you to engage your muscles to keep yourself balanced there are other items that you can use to keep yourself moving at your desk. We have discussed having grip trainers that you can squeeze from time to time to increase movements but there is another product you can purchase that can get you moving while sitting at your desk. Desk peddles or desk elliptical are small versions of stationary bikes or elliptical that you can place under your desk and use anytime while you are sitting. These can usually be picked up at a local store or bought online for anywhere from 20 dollars to several hundred depending on brand and or quality. The idea is simple, place the peddler under your desk and while you are at work just peddle. You will be moving your legs and getting your heart rate up a little during the day. You will also be burning extra calories that you otherwise would not be burning. There will be some trial and error with using any desk exercise products. For the peddlers you might have to adjust how you are sitting so that you will have a free range of motion to peddle. This positon might not be one that you are able to stay in all day. Taking 5 to 10 minutes every hour to just peddle while you do tasks like reading emails or browsing the internet will add up. Think about it, in a standard 8 hour work day if you peddled for 12 minutes every hour then at the end of the day you will have increased your activity by a little over an hour and a half! In a week's time that is 8 extra hours of activity and in a month that adds up to 32 hours that you spent moving that you otherwise would not be! Keep in mind that you are at work so the peddling probably won't be vigorous enough to get you into your target heart rate zone but if you recall the section on NEAT every extra movement counts!

The last thing we will cover in this section is standing desks. I love the concept of standing desks. What I don't like is the price tag that comes with them! There seems to be a few options, spend a lot of money on a standing desk that can raise and lower so you can stand when you want or sit when you need to. Or use a standing desk that is always up and then you do not have the option to sit. Others I know have placed stacks of books or boxes under their computer to raise it up so they can stand. I avoid this because I don't like the idea of my work computer, which I do not own, being placed on something that might be unstable. The truth is that standing at work can help boost productivity, help your post meal blood sugar levels return to normal more quickly and burn extra calories (although the research is conflicting on just how many extra calories). This is a product you might want to try if the resources are available to you.

I highly encourage you check into the options that I have shown in this section if you are someone who finds themselves sitting for a good portion of their work day. You might be surprised just how much a little extra movement can really affect your life on a physical, mental and spiritual level!

48

Increasing your activity: At Home

In the last section we learned about a few strategies and products that you can use to increase your activity at work, I think I made it well known that you can get a lot of extra activity by using a desk peddler for a couple minutes an hour. Now what can you do when you are not at work or if you do not have a job where you sit often, what can you do at home? Much like the last section we have gone over a few of these strategies in prior sections. I feel it is necessary to cover them again because movement and activity is a great way to improve your health and boost your weight loss.

The important thing is to make some time for activity, if you have children take them out to play and play with them instead of just watching. Run around the yard or the park with them; go for family bike rides on the weekends, sled ride with them in the winter. If they are playing on the playground walk laps around the play area, getting your kids involved is a great way to stay motivated and teach them the importance of activity. Don't have any kids? Take the dog for a walk or a run in the evenings after work. Don't have a dog? Put your head phones in and go for a walk yourself, or recruit the neighbor(s).

Be active while you watch TV! I mentioned before about stretching during commercials, a desk peddler could come in handy at home too! Peddle during commercial breaks or during your favorite show. Per hour of TV there is an average of 16 minutes of commercials. If you peddled during the commercials that gives you 16 minutes of activity per hour extra that you usually did not get.

The honest truth is that I do not know your home life; these suggestions could be perfect for you or they might not work for you at all. This comes down to you and your choices. You know what you are capable of and you know what type of time you have and activity you have available to you. Getting in more activity throughout your day is important; how you do it is up to you! Have you already been making the changes in your life to be more active? Will you begin focusing on those changes now or become more serious about them? This is a process that takes your total commitment. Your health and wellness doesn't punch a clock at 8 am and out at 5 pm Monday through Friday. This is a 24/7 commitment to your new healthier life. Ask yourself have you fully committed? You have to be honest with yourself, are you doing what it takes?

49

Increasing your activity: During Travel

This section might apply to you often if you travel for work regularly or it might only apply to you occasionally. When we travel we are typically busy, and taking care of ourselves when we are traveling for work or vacation usually doesn't rank high on the list. However you should still take a little bit of time to make sure you are getting in at least some physical activity.

If you find yourself traveling for work often it can be very difficult to get activity in due to flights, driving time, and hotel stays. Many hotels have small gyms that are available to guest, but you might never know what you are going to get. Some I have seen are fully stocked with plenty of equipment and others have barely anything in them and I would say meet the most basic requirements to be considered a "gym". There are things you can still do to get your activity in. You just might need to be creative.

As you might have noticed I will always say go for a walk. It is the most basic of activities that you can do and for the most part anyone can do it. You might not be able to go far yet but you can keep trying. Walk through the hotel, walk outside, walk down the hall to the stairs and go up a flight then walk to the other end and go down a flight. Walk on the treadmill if the hotel has one. You can also use the swimming pool if they have one. Walk around in the pool, swim laps. Make what is available to you at the time work for your needs! There are also inexpensive products you can purchase and take with you that will allow you to exercise in your hotel room. Getting quality resistant bands would allow you to pack lightly and get a resistance workout on the go. The plus side to bringing your own resistance bands with you is that you would be able to plan out your activities for the night and make it part of your routine. These exercise resistant bands can be a great addition to your home routine as well.

If you find yourself on vacation, make some plans that include some sort of activity. Plan a hike, or go for that walk on the beach in the morning that you always tell yourself you want to do but never get around to it. Many vacation spots allow you to rent a bicycle to get around instead of driving everywhere. The point is that you need to keep your health and wellbeing a priority even when you are on the road or away for vacation.

50

Exercise Vocabulary

Let's take a break from me scolding you about making sure you fit physical activity into your day. Today will be a change of pace that I think will help you when going forward with your weight loss and activity goals. As I have stated many times now the idea of this book is to give you the basic knowledge and build up from there. By the time you are done reading this book I hope that you are either at your goal or have the knowledge to reach your goal. Part of this process will typically lead you to doing your own research and looking into other sources for exercise or fitness advice. What you might find is great advice but there could still be some words or terms that are foreign to you. This section I will try to briefly go over some of those terms.

The first term is Flexion. This is the process of bringing two body parts closer together. Think of it as you are flexing a muscle like your biceps. How do you flex your bicep? By bending at the elbow and brining your forearm towards your upper arm. You are performing flexion at the elbow joint. Next we have extension, which is the movement to increase space between two body parts. It is the opposite of flexion, for extension you could straighten your arm back out at the elbow joint. This increases the distance between your forearm and your upper arm. Those terms are easy enough, and I am sure you already had a solid understanding of them.

Adduction is a term you might not be familiar with but will see it in the description of exercises. This term refers to the action of moving a body part towards the center line of your body. Think of it this way, put both arms straight out to your side. Now by moving at only your shoulder joints bring you're your hands together out in front of your body. This is easy to remember because the term starts with "add", you can think of it as "adding" to your body because you are bringing your body parts to you, like you are adding them to your body. Finally we have the opposite of that, which is abduction. This is the process of moving a body part away from the center line of your body. For example if you lift your leg straight out to your side away from your body, you would be abducting at the hip joint.

When you have an understanding of the terms that are used when describing an exercise it will ensure that you are completing it properly. This means that you will get the most out of the exercise and reduce your risk of injury. Keep an eye out for these terms as you do your own research and as we move forward through this book!

51

Calorie Tip!

It is very common when people are trying to lose weight or become healthier that they try to change up their diets by eating salads. This is a great idea and I am sure that you have increased your salad consumption in the last 50 days. That being said where people tend to fail is that they only count the calories for the lettuce or they under estimate how much dressing they are actually eating. This can lead to over eating without even realizing it.

It is important that when you are counting your calories that you are counting everything! That means you are counting the ketchup you ate with your fish, or the light ranch you put on your salad, or the extra cheese that you added as well. These things might not contain a lot of calories but if you are regularly neglecting to count them they can add up quickly and quietly sabotage your progress! This calorie tip is going to focus on salad dressings.

Salad dressings come is a huge variety, some high in calories and fat others low in calories, it is important to read the nutritional labels! Just because it might say fat free doesn't mean that the other ingredients are any better. We spent a week reviewing what is in a nutritional label so you should be able to make a good choice when selecting a dressing. Like everything else that you consume it is important to watch your portion sizes, which by day 51 I hope that I am just preaching to the choir. However, have you ever really looked at a portion size of salad dressing? A serving size of a popular ranch dressing contains 140 calories. Want to take a guess as to the serving size? 2 table spoons! That is not a lot of dressing. I doubt that it would cover much of your salad. There is a good way though that you can reduce the amount of dressing that you eat while still getting the taste. Instead of dumping the dressing on the salad order it on the side. Then dip your fork in the dressing before you use it to grab the salad. This will give you the flavor while reducing the amount of it you consume!

It is always difficult to change your habits, but small changes can yield huge results. Think about the salads that you have eaten in the past or that you have consumed since starting this journey. Have you put more than 2 table spoons worth of dressing on the salad? Did you record it as the proper serving size, or did you likely underestimate how much you used? Give this strategy a try, it might help you to both reduce your calories consumed and allow you to more accurately record your daily calories. Keep in mind this strategy could work with your other dipping sauces! Measure out a serving size of ketchup and dip your fork in it before you eat your fries. Look for opportunities to reduce your extra calories by implementing strategies like this one where you can! Diet smarter not harder!

52

Set Backs Happen

Let's face it, setbacks happen. You are going to fall off of the horse from time to time, you are going to want to give up or you are going to go back to your old eating habits for a few days. You might not want to keep going with this. The point is, we are human and with that we are flawed. You are almost 2 months into this journey and many of you might have fallen off the horse a time or two already. Maybe you haven't yet but you have been close, or maybe you will in the future. The important thing to know is that if or when it happens you pick yourself back up and keep going. If you step away or have a slip up it is not the end of the world. Failure is nothing more than a new starting line.

What do you do if you fall off this new life style horse? First thing you need to do is remind yourself why you opened this book in the first place. No one is reading this book for entertainment; this book was picked up because you wanted to make a change. Whatever that reason was for the change it must have been strong. Focus on that reason let it light a fire under you like it once did. This will help to give you the motivation to start again. Only this time you won't be starting from square one. You will already have a knowledge and skill set to get you back on track to achieve what you want to achieve.

Maybe this journey was harder than you thought; maybe going it alone isn't right for you. Look for a wingman to help you out. They don't have to have the same goals as you but don't underestimate the power of influence someone else rooting for you will have. It is very important to remember that you will need to ease back into things. Let's say you were doing well with exercising but then you just fell out of it and it's been a few weeks now. Don't just jump right back into where you were. You need to start slow and rebuild to where you were. You will get back to where you use to be quickly but you need to give your body time to readjust to the activity levels again.

Finally look at your goals again. You set those goals knowing that you could achieve them. We spent time on how to create goals that were achievable. Focus on those goals, when you started this those were what you wanted. You know that you still want to achieve those goals. Get yourself back in the mindset you once were in, and go after it! Remember this section, mark it down. If you find yourself having a hard time come back here and reread it. Find your drive to keep going. You are stronger than you think, you got yourself into this situation and you are able to get yourself out.

53

Get a Buddy.

The importance of social support cannot be undersold. We all need support at some point in our lives and at this point in your life you are trying to make some big changes. It can be very hard, and going at it alone can make it even harder. That is why you should consider getting yourself a good diet/workout buddy. Someone who will be able to relate to what you are going through. Someone who you will be able to receive advice from and someone you can bounce ideas off of.

This person could be your spouse or your current boyfriend/girlfriend. Find someone that you don't mind sharing detail of your life with. Your buddy could be your neighbor, a family member, or someone you work with. They don't have to have the same goals as you or the same workout and diet strategy as you. They don't even need to be in the same starting place as you. The key is to find someone who will help support you as you make these changes in your life.

You might be wondering if it can be so helpful for you to find a buddy then why am I waiting until day 53 to suggest the idea? Well simply put, I wanted you to focus on the information that was presented to you so far in this book. How often have you heard diet or exercise advice from another person or in some form of media? How many times have you seen the new miracle apple cider vinegar drink on Facebook that is supposed to help you lose all of your fat in 3 days? The point is that I wanted you to be building up your knowledge and applying it before you might develop a close relationship with someone on this life style change. If you have been following along and making these small changes to your life style then you are likely starting to see results. I felt it was important for you to begin applying the principles you have learned to your life and to see success without the influence of another person who might sway you towards a gimmick diet or a get fit quick plan.

That being said; consider finding a partner to join you. Make sure you select someone who will help you develop a positive relationship. It is ok to be a little selfish in this process. You need to find someone that will help you and someone you will be able to help. If you select someone and the relationship is all one sided, meaning that you have to always help them or they always have to help you without any return then the relationship might break down. There will be a need for a little give and take, and at times you might need someone who can be brutally honest with you. Take some time to consider if you would like to have a buddy join you and if so take even more time selecting someone. It could just help!

54

Nutrition: Sodium

It is time for us to tackle the big bad boogey man, sodium. We have all heard how sodium can cause all sorts of ailments, including high blood pressure, heart problems and kidney issues. What makes it cause all of these problems? How much sodium is too much, too little? Is sodium just a fancier word for salt? This section we are going to dive in and try to answer these questions, so you can make good choices about sodium consumption going forward.

To start, what is sodium? It is a mineral that is found naturally in our foods. As we learned in the section on minerals, plants absorb minerals through the ground and the minerals are then transferred and absorbed by those that consume the plants. However like other minerals sodium is added to packaged and prepared foods, in fact 75 percent of the sodium that we consume comes from processed food. These foods are things like lunch meats, pre made frozen meals, canned soups and so on. When it comes to sodium consumption you need to check the nutritional labels! The truth is that sodium has a great many uses as a food additive. It is a preservative, flavor enhancer, thickener, as well as many other uses. It is easy to see why it is added to so many foods!

Is sodium just another name for salt? The two words do seem to get used as the same thing when it comes to nutrition. That does not mean that they are in fact identical. As we went over sodium is a mineral, and salt is the common name for the chemical sodium chloride. In short salt is made up of 40 percent sodium and 60 percent chloride, so it is not straight sodium. So adding salt to your foods won't hurt you, right?

Since salt is not majority sodium and we get about three quarters of our daily sodium needs from other foods, then can we add it to our foods right? The answer is yes and no, but mostly no. Regular table salt has 25% of your daily recommendations per serving. The key is how much is a serving of table salt? It is smaller than you might be thinking! A serving of table salt is ¼ teaspoon! When you are done with today's reading go to your kitchen and measure out a full teaspoon of salt. That single teaspoon of salt equals your total daily recommendation of sodium! Now think about your eating habits, do you use that much salt during the day? If you do then you, like most Americans are consuming over your daily recommended limit.

Sodium is measured on nutritional labels in milligrams, which is a very small unit of measurement. Because the unit of measurement is so small the recommended daily value seems like a large number. You should aim to consume less than 2,300 milligrams of sodium a day. This includes the sodium that is contained in the food you eat as well as the salt you add to your food. When it comes to sodium the recommended daily amount is the upper end and you should try not to exceed that amount. However the average American exceeds the 2,300 milligrams a day by consuming 3,400 milligrams a day. That's more than 1,000 milligrams over what the maximum should be for the day!

What is the harm in exceeding your daily recommended amount? First let's start this by stating that sodium is an essential mineral, this means that the body has to have sodium to function! Sodium helps to keep our nerves and muscles working properly as well as fluid balancing. However consuming to much can have negative effects on your body!

Sodium attracts water, and when your diet is rich in sodium water is drawn into your blood stream. This causes the volume of blood to rise which in turn causes your blood pressure to rise. This is known as hypertension, and it can hurt your circulatory system in two main ways. First it causes your heart to work harder per pump; added strain on your heart in this form can cause damage. Secondly the increase in blood pressure puts strain on the walls of your arteries and organs. Prolonged high blood pressure can increase your risk of heart attack, stroke, heart failure, blindness and kidney disease.

So now we know that sodium attracts water, what organs have we touched on so far filter and use water? Our kidneys! The kidneys use sodium and potassium to control the process of moving water from the blood to the bladder. This is a process known as osmosis where a delicate balance of sodium is used to pull water across the cell walls of the blood stream into the collecting channels in the kidneys. The extra fluid that is stored in the bloodstream due to the high sodium levels means that the kidneys are put under extra strain that can damage the blood vessels that lead to the kidneys. If left untreated this could lead to kidney failure!

You have been tracking your food intake for a while now, and might have already been checking the amount of sodium you consume. Sodium is needed and unavoidable, but reducing the amount in your diet to be at or below the recommended daily amount can help reduce your risk of developing life threatening conditions. Take a moment to look at the food you are consuming, do you consume more than 2,300 milligrams a day?

55

How to Snack

We are all guilty of snacking. Snacking has developed a label of a big no-no in the diet community. However is it really that bad for you? Ready for a vague answer that I will try to expand on? The answer is yes and no. It really depends on what you are eating, how much you are eating and how often you are snacking. We have been learning all about how to monitor your calories by reading food labels so if you are staying in your calories range then snacking isn't a bad thing. If you are exceeding your daily calorie goal or consuming food that are high in the undesirable nutrients then snacking can be bad for you.

You need to treat snacking just like you would a regular meal; look at the food label to see what is in the snack food, how many calories and what the serving size is. For a snack of chips a serving size is only 11 chips but contains 140 calories. That is not a great deal of calories but it is also not a great deal of chips. When you are snacking on something like a bag of chips it is very easy to eat well over a serving size, think when the last time you sat down with a bag of chips and only ate 11. Going for a healthier snack doesn't mean you can eat more either. A good example of this is trail mix. This snack has a variety of nuts and other ingredients and is commonly thought of as a healthy snack. The problem is that it might be better for you than a serving of chips but there is still 180 calories in a serving, and the serving is less than 1/3 cups. That can be as much as a large handful of trail mix.

Snacking can have benefits. It can be a way for you to get extra nutrients in to reach your daily needs, and more importantly in the realm of weight loss it can help reduce hunger cravings between meals. Reducing your hunger feelings in between meals can be a game changer to help keep you from over eating! So how can you snack correctly? Pick low calorie snacks such as fruits or vegetables, and be mindful of the calories and serving sizes of any dipping sauces you might use like ranch. If you are going to snack on something like chips, count out the number of servings you want to eat and put them in a bowl instead of eating out of the bag. Once you finish the bowl be done, this can reduce the risk of over eating and underestimating the total calories consumed. Research also shows that chewing your snacks slowly and more thoroughly can help to make you feel more full, helping you to not over snack and sabotage your daily calorie intake. If you are feeling hunger between meals planning out a healthy snack could help you to not feel so miserable between meals. Just make sure you are recording the calories in your daily totals. Remember a "healthy" snack doesn't mean you can over eat with it, a calorie is a calorie! Keep in mind you might feel better from a healthier snack though!

The Healthy Food Paradox

We touched on this topic heavily yesterday but I feel it is important enough to review it again. There is this myth that people either don't understand or chose to believe and that is that you can eat more of the healthy foods because well they are healthy. "Sure I over ate, but it was healthy stuff". At this point in the book you might be realizing just how silly this idea really is.

We started out this book by hitting the ground running on what a calorie is and what your body does with them. We have gone over the different nutrients you find in your foods as well as their pros and cons. So you have the understanding that your body doesn't treat healthy food calories any different than unhealthy calories. However where I believe this idea that you can over eat healthy calories keeps persisting is the concept that not all calories are equal when looking at the nutrients. As we have learned this is true. When it comes to meeting your daily recommended nutritional values healthy foods will aid you in this. However a calorie is still a calorie so over eating healthy foods will have the same result as over eating unhealthy foods, weight gain.

Don't fall for this myth that you over ate but it's not that bad because at least it was healthy foods. Over eating is over eating. If you keep track of your calories, portion sizes, and daily Nutritional values then you will see success in your weight loss. Over eating will lead you back to weight gain and undermine your hard work. Over eating is over eating no matter what form the food takes.

Meal Prep

Following in line with our current theme of monitoring your calories and snacking we will be talking about meal prepping. When you hear the term "meal prepping" body building probably comes to mind. There is a reason for this, body builders typically need to consume a large amount of calories and watch their macronutrients to achieve their best results. A body builder will make up their meals ahead of time so that they know exactly how many calories they are eating during the day. This ensures that they are able to meet their high calorie needs. If meal prepping can ensure that someone is able to meet a high calorie intake then the same principle can be applied to trying to reach a lower calorie intake.

Meal prepping is something that takes time and as the name implies preparation. You need to plan out your meals ahead of time, buy the food and cook the food. Then you need to store the food until you are ready to eat it. This can be easy or complicated depending on what your goals are. Food prep can also take many forms. Some people will cook all of their lunches for the week on the weekend then store them in Tupperware to be heated up and eaten later. Some people will take the time to slice up a low calorie lunch of fruits and veggies before they leave for work in the morning. Many chose to measure out their dinner and place it in the slow cooker to be eaten for dinner when they get home. The key is that you have to find a strategy of meal prepping that works for you. There are hundreds of meals and strategies you can find online.

How can meal prepping help us lose weight? Prepping your meals ahead of time means that you know exactly how many calories you are going to eat for breakfast lunch and dinner. If you know how many calories you are going to eat ahead of time then you are less likely to take guess and eat too many calories throughout the day. For example let's say that I am on a daily calorie goal of 1500 calories. For breakfast let's assume I eat 300 calories and for lunch I eat 500 calories. That means that I have a remainder of 700 calories for snacks and dinner. Now if I preplanned my dinner and I know that it will be 500 calories, then I will have 200 calories left for the day. This means I can have an afternoon snack or a bedtime snack that day. Knowing how many calories you are going to have for each meal preplanned means you will not be caught off guard and come up short or over your daily goal.

Take some time to determine if meal prepping could help you. Start small and try prepping your lunches and snacks. Then add in other meals. It could help give you an edge in your weight loss journey by allowing for a more accurate calorie count because your meals are already pre measured and pre portioned out. Meal planning removes the guessing about how much space you have left in your daily calorie goal because you already know ahead of time!

58

No Pain No Gain Myth

The phrase no pain no gain can have serval different meanings. Often times you will hear people use it in the context that anything worth having is not going to be easy. That is not the context that I am claiming is a myth. The myth that we will be dealing with today is that exercising has to hurt either during or after an activity or you weren't trying hard enough. This is a myth that continues to persist and it can lead to injury.

Now some soreness is to be expected after you exercise, you are working out muscles and causing them to fatigue. The point is that you should not be in a great deal of pain. This doesn't mean that you should not push yourself in a workout, in order for you to force your body to adapt and change you have to push yourself. You should not be pushing yourself to the point that the exercise will hurt and cause you to feel beat up for days on end. This myth keeps going because we have associated the pain with working hard.

The problem is that this association between pain and hard work can lead to intense prolonged muscle soreness following exercise. When this happens you might be too sore to work out again in the following days, which could set you back on your target goals. Another effect it might have is on your emotional wellbeing. If exercising results in pain and extreme discomfort you might become discouraged. Becoming discouraged can make it harder to commit to being more active and cause you to give up on it.

The key is to find a level of activity that pushes your body into some discomfort but not to the point of physical pain. For each person the level of activity to push them to the point of physical pain is different. We have covered easing into exercise earlier in this book. Allowing yourself to ease into a workout or activity gives your body time to adjust as well as allow you to find that line between pushing yourself in a workout to an appropriate level or pushing yourself to physical pain. Becoming fit is a long journey; you do not have to be in a rush to go hard in your workouts! This is a marathon not a sprint, take a little time and build into it. After each workout go a little harder and a little harder. Within time you will be at a level that pushes your body to change and meet the demands you are placing on it.

59

Muscles of the Body: Core

In the various exercises we have covered in this book so far I have referenced your core muscles. What are the muscles that make up our core? What purpose do they serve? You might be surprised just how many muscles make up your "core" and how much they are involved in our daily movements.

When we discuss the core muscles we are talking about the muscles around your midsection. This includes the muscles on the front, sides, and back of your body. Commonly they can be referred to as your abs. The first muscle is the Rectus Abdominis, which is the most well-known muscle that makes up your "abs". This is the "6 pack" muscles that cover the front of your midsection. Next is the transverse abdominis, which is the muscle group that stabilizes the spine. Up next is the Internal and external obliques which help us to bend and twist at the waist. These muscles are located on the side of the body. The Erector Spinae and the Multifidus are used to stabilize the spine and individual vertebrae. The last of the main core muscles is a group called the Hip Flexors, which allows the upper leg to flex and adduct. There are many more but we are not going to get into every single muscle.

These muscles help to stabilize our upper body and pelvis (hips) when we are moving. They can also apply internal pressure to aid in expelling things from the body through breathing, vomiting, and defecation. The core muscles help us to align the spine, ribs and hips of your body to resist forces applied to it when you are both moving and remaining stationary. So as you can imagine they are very important during any and all movement that requires us to maintain balance.

You might have already noticed that with your increase in physical activity your core muscles might have felt sore, even if you didn't think you were directly working them out. The more active you are the more your core muscles are recruited for balance. As your body adjusts to this increase need in balance your core muscles will increase both in muscle strength and muscle endurance. We will be covering exercises that you can use to directly target your core muscle later in this book. Just hang in there!

60

Habits Taking Hold

We need to start today by acknowledging something big, you are now at your 60 day mark! This means that you have been reading and taking steps towards a healthier you for 2 months, plus or minus a day or 2. This is a big achievement, not only because you should be feeling positives from the changes you have made but because those changes will have begun to take hold as your regular daily habits.

There has been a myth out there that has floated around since the 1950's that says it takes 21 days for a new habit to become an automatic habit. This can be true for some people, and many of you reading this book might have found that 21 days was enough; others might have struggled longer or are still struggling with the new habits. I mentioned in an earlier section that the research shows that it takes on average around 60 days for new habits to become automatic. According to the research conducted by the "University College of London" it takes 66 days for a newly created habit to become second nature. Let's take a moment and define what a habit really is. The dictionary definition is "a settled or regular tendency or practice, especially one that is hard to give up." A better working definition is some action or behavior that is completed automatically.

Why is this important to know? The purpose of this book is to help you make a life style change, which I have stated numerous times. The changes you make need to become things that you automatically do so that the change is lasting. If the change is not lasting then you will fall back into a system of yo-yo and crash dieting again. Making your new habits concrete is the key to long term success. We are now at the 60 day mark and you have been working on making changes in your life, some of those changes might have been made 50 days ago, 23 days ago, or 3 days ago. You will make changes to your habits in the months or years to come. Breaking old habits is very difficult, and replacing them with new habits is even harder. You might become discouraged with the process and think "is it ever going to get easier?" The answer is yes, for the average person reading this your new habits should start to become second nature to you.

This section is in here because I wanted to remind you that change does not happen overnight. You did not hit your starting weight overnight; you did not develop the bad habits that gained you the weight overnight. The new habits will not take hold overnight. You need to be persistent and continue to push forward. Making changes is hard in the short term, but think to yourself how quickly the last 2 months have gone. The next several months will pass just as quickly. Stay motivated, keep the positive changes going, and before you know it those changes will not be changes anymore, they will be a part of you.

61

Sugar

It is time to tackle one of the big bad boogeymen of the health world! The dreaded sugar monster has been making people fat and ruining their lives for decades. Well not so fast. This section should not really come as a surprise to you at this point in the book. We know that we get the majority of our energy from carbohydrates and carbohydrates just breakdown into sugars. Those sugars are used to run the various systems of our bodies. So we need sugars in our diets, however there is a point where it can be a detriment to your health and wellbeing.

Like always it is time to learn a little about sugar so you can better understand its use and how much we should consume. For this section and throughout most of the diet/health community when sugar is mentioned we are talking about added sugar. Thanks to a recent change in the FDA rules on nutritional labels companies now have to put the amount of "added sugar" on our food labels. This is helpful for tracking your daily sugar intake and making sure, like the other nutrients you are not under consuming or over consuming but staying in that Goldie Locks zone of just right. On an ingredients label you might see the different names for sugar appear. Much like carbohydrates, sugars chemical name can change due to different types of molecular structures and where the sugar is derived from. The main ones we usually see are Fructose, Glucose, and Sucrose.

Typically if the word ends in "ose" it is going to be a form of a sugar. Example is lactose which is the naturally occurring sugar that you find in milk. Let's begin with fructose, which is a naturally occurring sugar found in fruits, some root vegetables, cane sugar and honey. It is also the sweetest of all of the sugars. Due to its sweetness it is one of the main components of high fructose corn syrups (the name kind of gives that away), and is a component of table sugar. Glucose is something we already have discussed in prior sections. This is the form that most carbohydrates are broken down into. Furthermore you might hear glucose be called dextrose. This sugar occurs naturally in fruits and plants because it is the primary product of photosynthesis, which is the process of plants converting light energy into chemical energy. Finally sucrose is found in sugarcane and the roots of sugar beets. Sucrose is actually formed when a molecule of glucose and a molecule of fructose join.

Now that we know what some of the basic sugars are; we are going to get down to some of the important nutritional information surrounding sugar, specifically added sugars. I am sure that you have heard all about how sugar makes you fat but does it really? What have we learned about fat so far? Fat is the body's way of storing extra calories that we consume no matter where those extra calories came from. For your average table sugar there are 16 calories per serving, and a serving size is 1 teaspoon or 4 grams. That is not a lot of sugar and works out to be just under 50 calories in a table spoon (12 grams). What we have learned so far, overeating by a little can add up to a lot in a couple of months or a couple of years. So eating more sugar than you need is a way to ensure you are consuming too many calories and gaining fat. However it is not likely that sugar is the sole culprit or the weight gain villain that it is made out to be. Yes adding that extra spoonful of sugar to your tea or coffee is going to increase the calories and every calorie counts we are going to focus a little on the calorie content of sugar but more on the health issues consuming too much can cause.

According to the World Health Organization 5 to 10 percent of your daily calories should come from sugar which for a 2,000 calorie a day diet means about 30 to 50 grams of sugar. The average American consumes about 13 percent of their daily calories through added sugar. That might not sound like too much over the recommendation but an average American does not eat only 2,000 calories a day. In fact some estimates put the average number of calories in the ball park of 3,500 calories a day! So let's look at it this way, if you get 10 percent of your daily 2,000 calories from added sugar that's 200 calories or 12.5 teaspoon of sugar or 50 grams of sugar. Now let's look at it with the calorie intake of 3,500. 10 percent of 3,500 calories is 350 calories from sugar or 88 grams of sugar. This is all assuming that the average person stays in their daily value of sugar range. We already know that the average American gets 13 percent of their daily calories from sugar and their average intake of calories is around 3,500 calories a day so let's figure it out with those two averages. 13 percent of 3,500 calories is 455 calories which works out to be 28 teaspoons of added sugar a day which is 113 grams of extra sugar a day. So that 13 percent for the average American turns out to be a lot more sugar than what it seems. The average American is consuming more than double the total grams per day than what is recommended.

What does this mean to our health? Well the possibility of weight gain is certainly there. The average American is over eating by 455 calories a day from sugar alone, but there is more to the health risks. Studies have linked excessive sugar consumption with an increased risk of heart disease. Think about that for a moment. We have already figured out that sugar can be adding to a person's weight control problems, but sugar in and of itself is not a sole driver of gaining weight. So it is possible for a "skinny" person to consume too much sugar and suffer the same consequences as those who are overweight. The studies found that a person who consumes on average more sugar than their daily recommendation was twice as likely to die of heart disease without any regard to the person's age, sex, and activity level or body composition. That is a big deal, we have gone over several of the ailments that come with being overweight or obese but consuming to much sugar regardless of other factors still increases your risk of heart disease.

Ok so we know that we need sugar in our lives, and we know how much sugar we should be consuming in a given day, 5-10 percent of our total calories. Now how do we watch out for the extra added sugars? Well it's both simple as well as misleading. Food labels now need to specify how much sugar has been added to a food that we eat. Where the problem comes up is that sugar is considered on a food label as being natural or added. Both are sugar but there can be differences. Sugar from an orange comes with natural sugars and fiber. We know that fiber helps to slow down digestion making us feel fuller longer and helps for sugar to be gradually released into the blood stream. So sugar from an orange is better than the sugar from orange juice. Although the orange juice might state that it does not have added sugars. That does not mean that your body will handle it as well as getting it from the orange fruit. Fruit juices typically remove the fiber which means that the sugars will be quickly released into your blood stream causing a blood sugar spike and sudden crash. We already covered the issues brought on by sudden blood sugar spikes so no need to cover them again here. On the nutritional label of fruit juices it might say that there is no added sugar, which can be misleading because there are natural sugars in the juice itself that might not be accounted for on the labels. Looking at a can of soda it can be easy to see the total added sugar; the average cola has 10 teaspoons per can. That means in a single can or regular cola you could be reaching your daily sugar needs!

To stay on top of your sugar intake you need to pay attention to your food labels and especially the drinks you consume. We discussed the "healthy food paradox" a few sections ago. Remember just because you are consuming the sugar from something "healthy" doesn't mean that it is any better for you than if you consumed the sugar in a can of soda. You have the skills and the knowledge to make wise choices when it comes to your dietary needs and goals. Keep tracking what you are consuming and be specific with everything! All of your actions and knowledge will add up to long term success.

62

Soda

Soda is one of those things that most Americans consume without ever giving it a second thought. We drink it with our meals, while we are out and about, when we need a quick pick me up. For most people it's a nice flavored drink that they enjoy. Now is the time for me to ruin it for you soda lovers out there.

Yesterday we learned about sugar and how the average American consumes too much. At this point in this journey you have been making changes to your diet. You have been cutting back on you calories consumed and I am sure as a result the soda drinkers reading this have severally reduced their soda intake due to the extra calories contained in the sugary beverages. I am sure though that there are still many of you reading this section who have continued to drink your daily soda. I get it, we all have our vices out there and maybe you're not ready to cut soda out altogether. It is time to take a look at just what happens when you consume soda regularly.

The average American consumes around 45 gallons of soda a year! That is a hefty amount, which adds up to just fewer than 500 cans in a year. According to the New York City Health Department drinking 1 can of soda everyday over the course of a year will account for an extra 50 pounds of sugar! That's not counting the extra sugar put in your coffee or the sugar that you add to your foods. That is 50 pounds of sugar a year just from drinking an average of a single soda a day! Let's take that a step further; breaking down those 50 pounds over the year into a monthly amount equals a little over 4 pounds of sugar a month! A single can of soda a day adds up to 54,750 extra calories a year which works out to be almost 16 pounds worth of fat! All of that from a single soda a day on average!

For some of you cutting out soda might have been all you needed to reduce your calorie counts. For others reading this, it might have just been one of the contributing factors to your weight gain. However the effects of consuming that much soda can be felt well past the possibility of weight gain. Studies show that consuming 1 to 2 cans of soda a day increased the risk of developing type 2 diabetes by 26 percent. Another study that followed 40,000 men for two decades found averaging a single soda a day increased your risk of heart attack by 20 percent, similar results were found for women.

The goal of this section is not to scare you into removing all soda from your life. If you enjoy soda you can have it, but moderation is the key. Consuming it too often increases your calories consumed and your sugar consumption. Be sure to account for both when adding it to your diet. Remember the goal is to become a healthier person by the end of this book!

63

Fruit juices

It should go without saying now that fruit juices contain a large amount of sugars. During the sugar unit we touched briefly on the sugar content in juices and if they were really any better than other sugary types of drinks. The truth is that in your natural fruit juices you will get vitamins and minerals as well as other nutrient not found in your soda style drinks. However remember the section on the "healthy food paradox"?

Fruit juices have long held the privilege of being assumed healthy; it's just fruit after all, right? Many fruit juices have added sugars and other ingredients that reduce their "healthiness". That's not to say that fruit juice is not a healthy alternative to soda, but when we are looking at it in the form of a balanced diet and weight management then fruit juice can be equal or worse than sodas. The average fruit juice has a concentration of 45 grams of fructose per liter which is only slightly less than the average for soda which is 50 grams per liter. Fruit juices can have a wide range of calories as well; your average apple juice contains 110 calories, where the average grape juice is around 150 calories. We know how much calories can add up over a period of time and contribute to a slow steady weight gain.

Fruit juices can contain the same amount of sugar as soda as well as the same calorie count. This means that replacing soda with a fruit juice really is only "trading the evil you know". As with many things that we have covered you need to be monitoring you calorie intake and following your daily recommended values. Fruit juices are high in nutrients but when coupled with the other foods that you consume during the day you might exceed your daily sugar values. With that you could be increasing your risk of type 2 diabetes and heart disease, even though you are consuming a "healthier beverage".

64

Diet Sodas

We have finally arrived at diet sodas, I am sure this is something that you might have seen coming or even have been eagerly waiting for. Maybe you haven't been waiting for this section, maybe you have switched to diet sodas due to their lack of sugars and no calories. You might have been considering a switch to diet sodas following what we have learned in the previous sections. Now we are going to dive into what the research shows us and find out if diet sodas are better for you than regular soda. Or could they be worse?

Many people opt to switch to diet soda as a way to reduce their calorie intake and reduce their sugar consumption. It is not a bad thought; you get to keep the flavor and carbonation of soda without those pesky unhealthy side effects. As you have probably notice there tends to be a theme with a lot of the food products that we cover in these pages, usually if it's being posed as something too good to be true then it likely is. The truth is that soda can be a big contributor to obesity and the metabolic syndrome that include things like high blood pressure, excess belly fat, high blood sugar and issues with cholesterol. Without the invention of diet sodas a few decades ago then the possibility that we would have a bigger obesity epidemic on our hands could be true. However that doesn't mean that there are not negative consequences that research into diet sodas is uncovering.

Diet drinks use artificial sweeteners that contain no calories so the assumption is that they are better than the calorie ridden sugar of regular drinks. This is true, artificial sweeteners do not contain any calories; however they are more sweet than sugar. Due to this increase in sweetness artificial sweeteners could stimulate a desire in you to want to consume more sugar. Think of it like a drug, the sweeter it is the more sweets you're going to want. Basically sodas that use artificial sweeteners might increase your desire for other sweets, and this could make a transition to a healthier life style more difficult. You are trying to eat healthier but your body desires more and more sugar causing an increase in cravings that you have to overcome.

Another study conducted on mice found that consuming artificial sweeteners could affect the bacteria in your gut, simply known as gut bacteria. Our digestive track is aided by bacteria that help to break down carbohydrates in our foods into sugars to be absorbed into the blood stream. Our digestive tracks are not perfect and do not completely break down all of the food we consume, which means that we pass it in our waste. If the food is not broken down and passes out of us that means that a certain amount of calories we eat are never actually absorbed by our bodies. What does this have to do with artificial sweeteners and bacteria? Well quite a lot it would seem. When the mice were fed the artificial sweeteners there was a change in their gut bacteria. The amount of bacteria that breaks down carbohydrates increased, which in turn meant that more calories were being broken down and absorbed into the body. This also caused an increase in the mice's blood sugar levels. This was then tested on a small group of humans who did not regularly consume artificial sweeteners. The results showed that within a week half of the participants developed changes in their gut bacteria and higher blood sugar.

Is this a nail in the coffin when it comes to sodas both regular and diet? No, but it should have you considering alternatives to soft drinks. The occasional soda will not kill you but you could be causing yourself to work harder at weight loss and switching to a healthier life style. Consuming regular soda increases your sugar intake and calorie intake. Drinking diet soda might reduce the number of calories that you get from your beverages but it could be causing you to absorb more calories from the foods you do eat. There can also be an increase in cravings for sugar and an increase in blood sugar levels associated with artificial sweeteners found in diet sodas. All of this could add up to sabotaging your attempts at this healthy life style change.

65

Moderation

Let's face it; there are a lot of negatives in this book. Whether intended to be or not a lot of what I have written has come across a little bleak. Just looking at what you have read over the last several days it could make it seem that everything that you drink that isn't water is slowly poisoning you and will send you to an early ailment ridden grave. Some of us are guilty of drinking too much soda, some of us didn't realize how much sugar we were really putting in our morning coffee, many of us might have thought we were making a good choice by switching to diet drinks.

In the health field there is a lot of doom and gloom. I feel that this is mostly due to the risks of harm our actions can have to our bodies. We only get one body and if we harm it with our health related decisions there might not be any way to correct course. For some of you who have struggled with weight management your whole life I am sure you have heard many of the things that are covered in this book. "You're going to develop disease "X" if you don't stop doing "Y"!" What we have covered is true, consuming to much sugar increases your risk of heart disease and type 2 diabetes, becoming obese could increase your risk of cancers and other ailments, and so on. Reading through this book where I lay out the risks associated with several behaviors and different food choices you might be starting to think that you need to cut everything out or you're going to die from some terrible disease.

You need to think of it like this, my goal is not to frighten you into adopting a heathy life style but to show you the consequences of regular abuse of certain things. Will a single cigarette give you lung cancer? No. Will a single can of soda or fast food burger give you diabetes? No. However years of smoking increases your chances of lung cancer just as years of fast food and soda increases your risk of diabetes, obesity, and heart disease. When we talk about the increased risk associated with certain behaviors like being sedentary we are talking over the long term. This is where the idea of moderation comes in.

I never tell people who come to me for advice to cut out everything that could cause them an increased risk of something. I tell them to consume things in moderation. If you like fast food cheese burgers you can still eat them, just don't eat them several times a week. Once a week, or a couple of times a month won't hurt you as long as you're accounting for it in your daily calories. You like sitting down and binge watching your favorite show? That's fine but don't make it a habit to do it every weekend. We all have foods we like and activities we enjoy that we know are bad for us. Cutting them out completely means you're going to miss them, and you could end up making yourself miserable. If you are miserable then the changes you make to improve your life will not last. Take time to do what you like even if it is bad for you, just do it in moderation. This will make it so that you are happy within your life style and decrease the likelihood of you to giving up and reverting back to old habits.

Moderation could be the key to keeping you motivated on this journey. In a prior section we spoke about being careful with rewarding yourself. Eating that burger or drinking that drink because "you earned it from that workout" will sabotage what you have achieved. That being said it is important to still allow yourself some of the pleasures you enjoy or you might find yourself giving up. Have that soda with lunch once or twice this week, not every day. Sit down and watch all 12 episodes of that show next weekend but not every weekend. Account for your actions and ensure that the good vastly out weigh the bad. Doing this will lead you to long term success.

66

Coffee

Please don't freak out and throw this book away as soon as you see the title of today's section. I say this, because have you ever told someone who is an adamant coffee drinker to not drink it? If you have then you have probably had to run for fear of them attacking you. Yes there has been a theme of the last several sections about drinks all having negative effects on our lives. Does coffee fall into that category though?

Coffee is one of those things that the health community has flipped flopped on more than a career politician in an election year. One year coffee is killing you and the next it is the only thing that's keeping your 90 year old grandmother alive. So where does the current science land on the issue? Well the World Health Organization has removed coffee from its list of foods that are potentially carcinogens. Some research suggests that it is actually good for you and could reduce the risk of several issues and diseases that we have covered in this book. However the reason for these potential positives to drinking coffee is unknown at this point in time. This doesn't mean that there are not studies that show an increase risk of certain cancers and cardiovascular diseases from regularly consuming coffee. So coffee could be good, or it could be bad. I am going to take a moment and do something that I have tried my best to leave out of this book, giving my personal opinion.

To me there are a few things that come into play with coffee and their potential positive or negative effects on your life. The chances are that when researchers are testing coffee they are probably testing straight black coffee. That means no sweeteners, no creams, and no other additives. Why is this important to consider? Think for a moment about what we have learned about sugars, calories, and other things that could be added to your coffee. Drinking straight coffee very well might be good for you but if you smother it in sugar, heavy cream, and other things that add to the calorie count then it is no longer good for you. How beneficial coffee is for you probably comes down to how you drink it. No matter how potential positive it might be for you, if you are drinking a coffee that has so much added to it that you're consuming 800 calories and 60 grams of sugar then it is bad for you.

I will let you make up your own mind on coffee. If you're not a coffee person then I do not see any reason to become one. If you are a coffee person I do not see any reason for you to give it up. At this point you have learned about the foods you eat, and you know if what you are adding to your coffee is doing more harm than good. What it comes down to is if you are consuming coffee then you need to be making sure that you are accounting for the calories and nutrients in it. Make sure it is fitting into your diet correctly and you will probably be just fine drinking it.

67

Super Food

I want you to take a second and think of what you consider a "super food". I bet that the first thing that came to mind was an avocado. Avocados are good in their own right; they have more potassium than a banana and are loaded with fiber and the healthy oils. However avocados are not the subject of today's topic. The "super food" we are going to discuss is the humble Kiwi.

That's right the little harry bright green kiwi fruit. There are far more benefits to adding a kiwi to your diets than what you might have ever thought. A kiwi has more potassium than a banana, is low in fats, high in fiber and has more vitamin C than an orange. Studies have shown that regular consumption of kiwi in our diets has several positive benefits. Vitamin C is necessary for skin health, and the abundance of vitamin C in the Kiwi can help to prevent damage caused by the sun and other pollutions. It might also help with overall skin texture. Some research even shows that kiwi consumption could aid in improving quality of sleep, as well as improvements in heart health. It could reduce your risk of kidney stones as well as lower your blood pressure.

This is a nice short section to give you some information on a food that you might have never really thought about. Today you should take some time and look into some other foods that you might enjoy or have neglected over the years. What nutrients they contain might surprise you. Some of what you thought were good could be bad and foods you might have neglected might be exactly what you need. Keep an open mind and do your research when you are looking to improve your diet. There is a whole world of foods out there, don't just settle for whatever the popular fad "super food" of the month is.

68

"Super Foods"

I gave you a really easy baby step into the world of super foods yesterday by introducing you to the nutritional benefits of kiwi. Does that make it a super food? No. Does the nutrient's found in avocados, beets, and kale makes them super foods? No. The idea behind "super foods" is that if you start eating them then you will start reaping all of these amazing benefits and you won't have to change your bad habits. "Why change my poor diet when I can just add a super food to it and that will balance it all out!"

It should come as no surprise to you that the idea of a single type of food is going to solve all of your problems is a lie. The problem though is that this is a comforting lie. "I ate an avocado with my lunch today so I can have that extra ice cream tonight". "I can put a lot of dressing on that my salad because it's kale and that's a super food". Does that sound ridiculous? Have you fallen for this comforting lie before? The truth is that the super food lie continues because it provides people with an excuse to take certain actions in their diet and exercise guilt free.

People tend to flock to foods like kale, avocados, pomegranates, goji berries, and so on because they think that it will offset their poor food choices. From what we have learned so far does that sound like it is going to work? That was an easy no wasn't it? Does this mean that those foods are not good for you? That's another no. I am not claiming that the foods that are generally referred to as super foods are not good sources of nutrients but what I am going to say is that they are not enough in and of themselves. We have learned about the importance of having a balanced diet. This means that you are meeting all of the daily values such as the daily value of fiber or daily value of protein. You cannot achieve all of your nutritional needs from a single type of food. The myth that follows super foods is that it is all you need to meet your nutritional requirements.

If you enjoy some of the foods that fall into the "super food" category by all means continue to incorporate them into your diets. The important thing to remember is that you do not rely solely on a single food to meet your nutritional need. Keep an open mind with your food choices, much like the kiwi in the last section you might be surprised by what you discover with other foods! Like always be sure that you are coupling your diet with your goals. If your goal is to lose weight, make sure that you are cutting calories but eating foods that will still meet your nutritional needs to prevent malnutrition.

69

Spot Targeted Weight Loss

One of the questions that I get most often is "how do I lose the fat from [insert body area here]?" Some people want to know how to lose belly fat, some want to know how to lose arm fat, or leg fat. What they are talking about is the idea of spot targeted weight loss. You see this often with people wanting to lose belly fat so they do ab workouts, or people want to lose that fat build up on the back of their arms so they do triceps exercises. The question is does this work?

The research leans heavily towards no. However there is some current research that shows that it might not be completely impossible to a degree. First let's look at how our body uses the fat for energy. Fat is formed from the extra calories we consume and is stored as triglycerides inside the fat cells. When our body calls on our fat stores for energy it cannot just take these triglycerides and burn them due to their inability to pass through the cell membranes. Special enzymes break down the triglycerides into free fatty acids and glycerol then release them into the blood stream to be used by the body for energy. This is really just a lot of words to say that fat is broken down and transported to where the energy is needed by the blood stream. So what could that tell us? Due to the fact that the energy from fat stores is delivered from the blood stream, which runs through the whole body, the fat being burned could be coming from anywhere.

Various studies have been done testing the idea of spot targeted weight loss, starting back in 1971 a study was conducted on the swinging arm of tennis players compared to their non-swinging arm. The idea was simple, if targeted weight loss was possible then it would show less fat in the swinging arm because it is used more often. The result showed that fat was equal in both arms, although the swinging arm did have greater muscle mass. Other studies have tested the idea with a more hands on approach where the participants were completing a weight training program where they only performed lifts with 1 leg for 12 weeks. In the end the results were no different from the other studies; fat content was equal for both the trained and untrained leg. The idea of spot specifics weight loss seems to be dead in the water.

There is a little bit of hope for the concept though! A 2017 study out of the *University of Rome* had participants split into two groups. One group did only upper body workouts while the other group did only lower body workout. The researchers also added in 30 minutes of light cycling immediately following the workouts for both groups. The results were very different from other studies! The group that trained upper body only lost a significant amount of fat from the upper body and a very small amount from the lower body. The lower body group had the exact opposite results, losing the vast majority of fat from the lower body and less from the upper body. Why might this have happened?

What we know is that when you use your muscles your body will increase blood flow to that muscle. This is often referred to as "a pump" in the lifting community. This happens because as you use your muscles they require more energy and produce more waste, so from what we have learned so far we know that the blood stream carries the energy to the muscles and the waste products away. It stands to reason that due to the increased blood flow to the muscle groups you are exercising the body might use the fat from that area as well.

Think for a moment though, why would this study show spot reduction is possible while the others did not? Well there could be a few things at play. First the participants exercised their whole upper or lower body, unlike the other studies that did just one specific limb. The bigger contributor to the results however was probably the 30 minutes of light cycling following the workout for both groups.

Looking at what we know so far, fat is broken down and shipped to the area that needs the energy. Energy that we do not use is turned into fat, so this means that the fat that we break down during the workout that is not used by our muscles will return to the fat cells to be stored again. When the 30 minutes of light cycling was introduced it is very likely that the activity was able to burn off the extra fat that was released into the blood stream. The cycling activity could have been light enough to not prompt the body to continue to release more energy from the fat stores and instead use what was still in the blood stream from the other exercise. This means that the fat was not returned to be stored for later use again and would account for the drastic difference in fat loss areas between the 2 groups.

The study shows that it might be somewhat possible to target fat loss in specific areas of the body to a degree. However the study is the only one of its kind right now and it used a small sample size. This means that there is a possibility of the results being a fluke, and we should wait for more studies to be completed before calling it a fact. That being said the science and reasoning behind the results does seem sound, but I still fall into the line of thinking that reducing calorie intake to a level 15-25% below you TDEE coupled with a whole body exercise program is the best method for fat loss. If you are someone who is struggling with a specific area then you might be able to give this a try for yourself. Follow the same guidelines of the study, perform the exercise on a specific region of the body and follow it up with 30 minutes of light cycling. It is possible that you could see some results.

70

Primary and Secondary Fat Sites

Continuing with the theme of fat I want to talk about primary and secondary sites. We have already touched on this way back towards the beginning of this book. The science shows that we store fat in specific areas first; these areas are called the primary sites. For women it is typically their butts and thighs and men it is our bellies. Secondary sites referrer to the other areas that we store fat, which basically means our face, arms, back and so on. It really boils down to the fact that we will store fat in certain places first then in other places throughout the body after the first places start to "fill up".

The concept of primary and secondary sites is why you typically will start to feel your pants getting a little tighter when you first start to gain weight. If you continue to gain then maybe your collar will begin to get a little tighter as you increase fat around your neck and face, then possibly down your arms. Everyone is different and unique; however fat storage locations are dictated by our hormones. For men testosterone tells your fat to go to your belly while estrogen tells women to store it in their legs and butts. As we age and our levels of these hormones decrease then the storage sites might change a little and begin to just spread throughout the body.

Do the areas that I described as primary sites match your "trouble areas" for weight loss? Men are you finding that your belly fat just wants to hang on until the bitter end and be the last to leave? Ladies do your thighs and butts just not want to shrink? Sure they might have shrunk a little with your weight loss but not as much as your face or arms and so on. This is because our bodies tend to follow a simple pattern for weight gain and weight loss. For most people the last place that you put the weight on is the first place you take the weight off of. Does that hold true for you? Maybe your neck or face thinned out before anywhere else on your body. Every time you lose some weight do people always comment that you lost it in a certain area?

Let's face it, this can be very frustrating because you might be losing all sorts of pounds on the scale but the inches around your belly or thighs just don't want to shrink. This is where you need to remain persistent. The fat around your "trouble spots" didn't get there overnight and it certainly won't come off overnight either. Imagine that your body has a check list as you lose weight. On this check list the secondary storage sites are given priority, and need to be cleared out before you get to the primary sites. Eventually you will work your way down that check list and that fat will be used but it just takes time. We learned in the last section that spot reduction could be possible but primary and secondary fat stores is sound science and something that is part of weight loss. Stay on this path and you will see the results you want!

71

The Dreaded Plateau

Anyone who has tried to lose weight has come across the weight loss plateau at some point. For those of you who are unsure what the plateau is, it is when you are having steady weight loss then suddenly weight loss stops. You didn't change your diet or activity level but for whatever reason you are no longer losing the weight. This is incredibly frustrating for people, you are doing everything that was working before and suddenly nothing is working anymore! Be honest, have you hit the plateau in the past and then gave up? Did you attribute the stall to something out of your control like the starvation mode myth?

We are covering this now because we are heading towards the middle of our third month, which means that many of you might be experiencing a plateau right now or in the near future. You likely found that when you started this adventure you were having great success early on, the calorie counting and portion control was working, exercising was becoming a habit that you enjoy and now it has come to a screeching halt. What causes a plateau? Honestly, there could be any number of factors. First you might be retaining water as your hormone levels adjust to your new weight. This is usually temporary and can result in a sudden rapid weight loss once the water weight is "released". Another possibility is that you have dropped enough weight that your TDEE is now to close to the amount of calories that you are consuming. We already know that as our bodies get smaller they require less calories to operate, so if you have dropped enough weight you might need to reassess your TDEE and calorie consumption to get back on track. There is another reason, one that you might not want to hear. It could be your fault. Think back on if you have been relaxing on your portion sizes or calories consumed. Are you eating more than you thought? Are you not exercising as much or as hard as you were? These are questions you need to answer honestly, and if you find that it is your fault then an easy correction can be made to get you back on track.

Just remember that plateaus are a part of weight loss, and don't let them get you discouraged. Typically they are short lived and you will be back on track in no time. If your plateau is lingering on for an extended period of time like a month or more then you might need to look into your calorie intake and your exercise program. Changes may need to be made to get you back on track! For me personally when someone encounters a plateau I advise them to not change any of their habits for 2-3 weeks. This gives your body time to adjust to your weight loss and it is possible that you will start losing weight again. If the plateau continues then you need to reassess what it is you are doing and take action with your calorie intake and exercise program to get the weight loss going again.

72

Types of Diets: Atkins

I have made my opinion on restrictive diets known pretty early on in this book. I am not a fan of them, I feel that they will work in the short term but will lead to periods of weight loss while you are on the diets and periods of weight gain when you are not on the diet. Changing your life style to being more active and improving your relationship with food will allow you to maintain the weight loss for the long term. All of that being said the whole goal of this book is to educate you on health and wellness and to set you up to make informed decisions on your weight control. Due to this I do not want to hide you away from the restrictive diets out there just because I disagree with them. For the next couple of days we will briefly review some of the types of diets out there and what they consist of.

Up first will be the "Atkins diet". The diet has been around since the 1970's and has evolved a little over the years. The creator Dr. Atkins believed that weight gain was the result of eating too many refined carbohydrates especially sugar. This goes in line with some of what we have covered already, but the Atkins diets allows you to eat as much protein and fat as you want. The whole point of the Atkins diet is to get your body into a state called ketosis, which is when your body doesn't have enough glucose and switches to fat for energy. Sounds great that instead of your body burning the carbohydrates that you eat, it is burning the fat that you have stored in your body. There are 4 phases to the diet where in phase one you cut almost all carbohydrates out of your diet, eating as few as 20 grams. In phase 2 you continue to eat only 12-15 grams of carbs a day while avoiding foods with added sugars. In phase 3 you gradually increase the range of foods that you eat and add around 10 grams of carbs back into your diet per week. The final phase is maintenance, where you met your goal weight and now maintain your diet for life.

What's really happening here is that carbs typically make up the majority of our calories consumed. It is likely that weight loss happens because restricting carbs will result in a reduction of calories. One of the problems with very low carb diets is that there can be side effects of not having enough sugar. People might experience headaches, dizziness, weakness, fatigue, constipation, and blackouts. Remember to always check with a doctor before beginning a diet program such as this one.

73

Types of Diets: Vegetarian

A vegetarian is not a short term restrictive diet, it is a life style. In this life style a person only eats fruits and vegetables. Although it is common for some vegetarians to eat fish or eggs the goal is typically to only eat plant based foods. As we have learned it is not a necessity to eat meats to get all of your nutrients, however remember that plant based proteins are known as incomplete, but it is possible to get all of the amino acids by consuming a variety of different plants. Therefore a vegetarian life style is one that can be maintained for a person's entire life.

The premise is very simple for the average vegetarian, if it is meat don't eat it. There are subsections of vegetarians such as Lacto-ovo-vegetarian; this group avoids animal meat as well as fish. Pescatarians will eat fish but not animal meat. Lacto-vegetarians will eat dairy products but won't eat eggs, and finally ovo-vegetarians will eat eggs but not dairy. That's a lot of options that you have to choose from, so if you are someone who thinks you would enjoy a vegetarian life style but don't want to give up all meat or dairy then there are options available. Remember your diet is your choice. If you want to eat mostly vegetarian but want the occasional burger then you can do that, just because you label yourself as something doesn't mean you are stuck in that group forever.

Vegetarian diets have been associated with a reduced risk of various conditions including diabetes, heart disease, obesity, and hyper tension. This is due in part to the dietary choices; the plant based foods are usually of the more healthy variety. Vegetarians usually consume less saturated and

Trans fat as well as less simple carbs. Another contributing factor could be that those who are more strictly involved with their dietary choices are more likely to pursue an active lifestyle as they tend to be more health conscientious.

There can also be risks associated with becoming a vegetarian. You might fail to get all of the vitamins and minerals needed through your plant based diet. We mentioned earlier that without consuming meats you are not getting the complete proteins your body needs. It is important for vegetarians ensure that they are consuming a variety of foods or they risk becoming malnourished. I personally enjoy vegetarian food options but I do not consider myself one. For me the diet I enjoy is a combination of plant based and meat options. If you are someone who is considering making the switch to a vegetarian diet ease into it, begin by slowly replacing your current meals with plant based ones over a period of time.

74

Types of Diets: Weight Watchers

I am sure that you have heard about the weight loss program called "Weight Watchers". It is the most popular weight loss program in the United States and has been around since the 60's. Millions of Americans have found success through this program; it has even become a favorite to recommend by doctors. What is the program and what makes it so popular?

The program is based on a point system. Different foods are allotted a different number of points. The points are dependent of the fat, sugar, and protein content of the foods we eat. The higher the protein content the lower the number of points gained, on the other side the higher the sugar content the more points gained. The idea behind the points is to change your dietary habits to be more fruit and vegetable based as well as lean protein and less fat or sugary food. Participants in the program are given a goal for points to reach per day. These points are based off how much the person weighs and what their weight loss goal is. It appears that the point system is designed in part to reduce your calories consumed by assigning higher point values to foods with higher calories.

There is a secondary component to the success of the Weight Watchers program and that is the community that they have built. The community is a group of people who are enrolled in the program and meet up to discuss their weight loss as well as provide support. Losing weight can be stressful and often you might feel like you are stuck out on your own little island dealing with all of the possible problems yourself. Becoming part of the weight loss community allows you to discuss what you are going through with people who are experiencing the same issues or who have managed to get passed them. Online meetings are also available to those who might not be able to attend in person meetings as well. Research has shown that people who were referred to Weight Watchers on average lost twice as much weight as those who tried standard programs over a 12 month period.

My opinion on the Weight Watchers program is that it can be successful for those who join and follow the guidelines. I think the point system is a clever way to get people to change their diets, much like I suggested earlier in this book. If a person is looking to lose weight through reducing calories you will naturally gravitate towards healthy low calorie options due to the increase in the volume of the foods compared to higher calorie options. The point system follows this same idea by awarding fewer points for low calorie options, the fewer points a food has the more of it you can eat. Finally I believe that the community aspect cannot be undersold. Having a support structure is very important and the program allows you to get in touch with others who are having the same experiences as you.

75

Types of Diets: South Beach

This diet plan has been around since the 90's but become popular after the book about the diet became a best seller in 2003. In all honesty this diet plan follows along with a lot of what we covered early on in this book. The difference is that it follows the same low carb idea that many diet plans use. You will notice this trend with a lot of diets because it is an attempt to get around having to count your calories. Remember high carb food options usually have high calorie content, and the majority of the calories we consume a day are from carbohydrates. It goes to reason that if you reduce your carbs you reduce your calories without having to actively count them.

The south beach diet however focuses on making the carbohydrates you eat come from things like whole grains and specific fruits and vegetables. This also goes in line with a lot of what we have covered. Remember there are simple and complex carbs and they can be broken down at different rates in the body. The more complex the carbohydrate is the longer you will feel full and the steadier your blood sugar levels will remain. This particular diet has 3 phases to it. In the first phase you will reduce your carbohydrate consumption in an attempt to balance out your blood sugar level. This usually lasts for around two weeks before moving into phase 2. In the next phase you slowly introduce carbohydrates in the form of fruits and vegetables. The idea is for the dieter to reintroduce the "good" carbs and limit the "bad" carbs. This phase 2 lasts until the participant meets their goal weight. Once you are at goal weight you adopt the lifestyle and attempt to make good food choices to maintain the weight loss for life.

Reading this you might be thinking that this is very similar to what you have learned so far in this book. As I stated earlier I tend to agree except for the lack of focus on calories. Reducing carbohydrates in your diet will typically result in lower calories consumed which in turn leads to weight loss. However it is an imperfect process. Lowering you carb intake will reduce calories but there is nothing stopping you from over eating the other nutrients. If you over eat in the other foods and exceed your calorie intake then you are going to stall your weight loss or gain it back. Because of this I will always support a lifestyle change focused on calorie and portion control. Knowing exactly what your body needs and exactly what you are putting into it allows for the most accurate weight management. The end game is the same however. The goal is to lead you to a position in your life that you have the knowledge on how to maintain your weight through a healthy diet that doesn't require meticulous monitoring of everything you consume.

76

Exercise: Crunches

The crunch is something that we have all done at some point in our lives. Maybe you love doing them but it is more likely that you hate them. The crunch as an exercise is a great way to target your core muscles most notably the rectus abdominis, also known as the 6 pack. When I say the word crunch what comes to mind? Often people envision lying on their backs with their hands on their necks trying to sit all the way up until their upper body is vertical. That exercise is known as a sit up and is very different from the crunch. In a sit up you are using your abdominal muscles to stabilize your core while you bend up at the waist. The actual action of bending up in a sit up is completed by using muscles know as hip flexors and not your abdominals. A crunch is very different; it involves contracting your rectus abdominis and bending your upper body forward at the spine.

How do you perform the crunch? First you need to lay down flat on your back bending your legs and placing your feet flat on the floor. You can move your feet closer or further from your body to find a comfortable position, keep in mind that typically the further from the body you move your feet the harder the exercise will become. At this point most people will place their hands behind their head and pull on their neck during the exercise. This is something you should avoid due to the increased risk of injury. My preferred method of hand placement is to place your palms flat on the ground to the sides of your body. Now you are in position to begin the exercise. Remember the goal of a crunch is not to bring your entire upper body up off the ground. Instead you will contract the abdominal muscles and curl up by bending at the spine. First your shoulders will leave the ground then focus on each vertebra in your back lifting up off the ground individually, starting at the top and working down your back. As you curl up slide your hands along the ground towards your heels. I like to use my heels as meter for how far I am going to curl up by trying to make contact with my heals through my fingers. The further out my feet are the further I need to curl up to reach them. You will complete the exercise when your shoulders are a few inches off the ground and your upper back is not contacting the ground.

Once you have reached the top of the exercise slowly lower yourself back down to the floor. If you want to get more out of the exercise do not lower yourself all the way back to the floor, try keeping your shoulder about an inch from the ground. This will keep your ab muscles tight and engaged; increasing their time under tension. This is a great exercise to perform if you wish to tighten up your core muscles. Be sure that you are focusing on curling up using only the rectus abdominis and not using momentum to go from the starting to the ending position. Now it's your turn to give it a try. Start out small with a couple sets of ten every day then increase the amount you do over time.

77

Energy Drinks

Millions of people turn to energy drinks to boost their energy throughout the day. We have all been there, didn't sleep well and need that boost in the morning. That tired feeling hits you like a ton of bricks around 2 in the afternoon. So you turn to an energy drink to give you a nice shot to finish out your day. Let's face it we all have those days that we are just not with it, and that caffeine jolt can help drag us across the finish line. If you are someone who drinks energy drinks regularly I am sure you have heard all of the risks and warnings from everyone around you, but are they right? Should you really avoid energy drinks?

To get to that answer I think we need to take a moment and go over some of what is in the drinks. The average 16 ounce can of energy drink contain 54 grams of sugar, which as we learned from the sugar unit is a lot! Keep in mind that the more sugar you consume the more your body has to produce insulin to deal with it. This action could eventually make you insulin resistant and lead you to being diabetic. The next major substance found energy drinks is caffeine which is measured in milligrams. On average energy drinks contain around 200 mg of caffeine; half of the daily recommendation of 400 mg. From looking at it the worst thing about an energy drink could be the sugar content and not the caffeine like most people would assume.

From a health standpoint it would seem that energy drinks could cause a spike in blood sugar that could lead you towards diabetes. If you are already at risk of diabetes from other conditions then consuming energy drinks regularly could increase your risk. There is a high amount of caffeine in the average energy drink, but for many people they could reach the same amount of caffeine in their coffee drinking habits. The area that I feel you need to be concerned with is the calorie content. Many energy drinks out there can have 200+ calories and when coupled with the increase in sugar consuming them regularly could be holding you back from reaching your health and wellness goals. Keep in mind that research from the American Heart Association found that drinking 1 to 3 energy drinks a day could disrupt your hearts rhythm. Although you might be able to work in the calorie allowance in your daily calorie needs you could be causing your heart extra unneeded stress.

78

Obesity: Fatty Liver Disease

Many people do not realize just how important your liver is to your health. Yes we have all heard about people needing liver transplants, but that's just for people who drink too much, right? Well, that can be true. People who consume alcohol regularly can develop the condition known as fatty liver disease, and in most cases it can be reversed with abstinence from alcohol. However poor diets and obesity can also develop fatty liver disease in a person. You read that correctly, a "skinny" person with a poor diet can develop the condition as well as those who are obese. However it is prevalent in the obese community due to the excess fat getting stored in the liver.

What is the liver? The liver can sometimes be referred to as the work horse of the body. It completes an array of tasks which include converting food into energy, processing fat in your blood, removing harmful toxins, and it even helps your blood to clot. We should strive to take good care of all our organs, looking at all of the work the liver does it might be one of the most important organs to keep in tip top shape. Now what is fatty liver disease? The classification we will be discussing in this section is called nonalcoholic fatty liver disease or NAFLD for short. It is diagnosed when a person's liver contains fat in more than 5% of the cells. It is becoming more common and currently effects 25% of American Adults. The bad, you might be asking; developing NAFLD can increase your risk of heart disease. If it is left untreated (such as remaining obese for years) it could cause the development of nonalcoholic steatohepatitis which could cause scaring on the liver increasing your risk of liver cancer.

As I mentioned you can develop fatty liver from other habits besides obesity, such as drinking heavily or keeping a poor diet. However excess weight seems to be the main culprit. Over the years the number of overweight and obese people has increased, and with that the number of people who have NAFLD has grown with them. This is thought to be a result of poor diets of regular processed foods and high amounts of carbohydrates and sugars. Sedentary life styles could also be a major contributor. A study conducted in October of 2017 looked at healthy men with low levels of liver fat and had them consume 650 calories from sugar daily for 12 weeks. The study found that they not only increased their liver fat but also changed how their bodies metabolized fat.

Luckily a person can generally reverse their NAFLD through proper diet and exercise. Some studies show that losing just 3% to 6% of your body weight could reduce the levels of fat in your liver by up to 40%. For many of you reading this you might have already lost that amount of your body weight. As long as you are making positive changes to your body weight, activity level, and diets then you will be making positive changes with your liver!

79

Muscles of the Body: Upper Back

The back is a complex system of muscles crisscrossing and connecting all over the place. You have your shoulders, spine, scapula, and neck all connected to a variety of muscles. In this section we are going to look at the some of the bigger muscles of the upper back and their importance to our health. These muscles include the trapezius, and latissimus dorsi.

The trapezius, traps for short, is a large fan shaped muscle that covers a large portion of the upper back and the back of the neck. Your body has two of these muscles that are symmetrical on the left and right and meet at the spine. The traps are responsible for moving, rotating, extending the neck, and stabilizing the shoulder blades. Next your latissimus dorsi, lat's for short, is one of the largest of the back. The lat's connect to your spine, pelvis, ribs, scapula, and upper arms. Like the traps you have two lat's, one for each side that are symmetrical. One of their main functions is to stabilize the back and surprisingly move the arms through adduction. Remember back to our vocabulary terms, adduction is when you bring your limbs towards the body. If you hold your arms straight out in front of you then pull your arms back towards you; this is adducting your arms, and your lat's are being used here.

It is no surprise that when people get into lifting weights and exercise they tend to gravitate to working out the muscle that you can see. These muscles are the arms, shoulders, and chest commonly, and the back usually gets forgotten. We just briefly reviewed two of the major muscles of the back and you could see how many different areas that those muscles connect too. When your back is weak or has a muscle imbalance it can affect our daily lives usually in the form of pain or discomfort. A weak trapezius could lead to neck pain as well as instability in the spinal column. Whereas weak lat's could cause shoulder pain. It is important to note that weakness in the back muscles is not the only thing that could be causing you pain, tightness could be a culprit as well. When the muscles of the back are tight or imbalanced then they could pull on the other parts of the body. If your traps are tight it could be possible that they will pull your spine or neck out of alignment, which in turn could cause you a great deal of pain. Tightness in the lat's could result in a pulling on the hips or shoulders, also leading to a miss alignment resulting in pain.

The moral of the story? Your back is an incredibly complex structure of muscles connecting all over the place. When you do not take the time to give your back a little attention things can weaken or be pulled out of alignment causing you a great deal of discomfort. If you are someone who experiences back or neck pain; like millions of Americans do, it might be worth it to add some back exercises and stretches to your daily routine. That never ending back pain you experience just might be alleviated with 5 minutes of daily stretching!

80

As Seen On TV: Ab Wheel

As seen on TV products are for the most part not the best exercise equipment out there. We spoke in an earlier section about quackery and how to spot it when looking at a product or claim. Often times you are able to see a large amount of quackery in as seen on TV exercise products. Does that mean that they are all bad?

The easy answer is no. There are some products out there that for sure work in the manner that they are intended to. One such product is the "Ab Wheel". This product has seemed to move away from it's as seen on TV roots and has found a home in many gym ab corners as well as in our homes. Let's start out with the basics, what is an Ab Wheel? You might have seen it called a variety of names but the common term in the fitness community is just simply an ab wheel. In its most basic form it is nothing more than a wheel with two handles on each side. There are more complex ones on the market that have multiple wheels or handles that you can also strap your feet into for a different style of exercise, but for this section we will just use the basic single wheel and two handle design.

Now that we know what it is how do we use it? The most basic use it relatively easy, well in theory that is; in practice the exercise can be very challenging. What you do is start on your knees with your hands on the handles and the ab wheel out in front of you. You now can lean out rolling the wheel out until you are in a position like you are on all fours with your arms straight beneath your chest and your back straight. To begin you will now start to lower yourself towards the ground by rolling the wheel out in front of you. As you do this you will extend at the hips and your shoulders will extend. Keep your back and arm muscle tight to remain balanced and controlled. You can lower yourself as far as you want, however for beginners you might not be able to go too far. Here is where the abdominal work really comes into play. Return yourself to the starting position by contracting your core abdominal muscle and "pull" yourself back up to the start. It is likely that you will feel this action working your abdominals, shoulders, back, and hip flexors as they all work to keep you balanced and return you to the starting position.

The benefits to this exercise can be pretty vast. It engages your arms, chest, back, core, and legs, but mostly focuses on your abdominal contractions. The equipment itself can be very cheap to purchase and the amount of space you need to perform the exercise is very small, making it ideal for a home use product. Some research has also shown that the engagement from the abdominal muscles is greater in an ab wheel exercise than the crunch. Everything sounds great doesn't it? You can get a great abdominal workout that also has the benefits of activating other major muscle groups of the body. It is a cheap piece of equipment that is available in most chain retailers or online. However there might be a few things to consider before attempting to use the product.

Full disclosure I have been using the ab wheel off and on since I was a little kid and my parents owned one. I have always found it to be a great workout and I credit it for the development of my abdominal muscles. All of that being said there are some draw backs to the product. First being that it is a hard workout! If you are new to the exercise or fitness in general you might get a nice serving of humble pie when you first try to use it. You might realize that your muscles are not as strong as you might have thought and you are not able to lower yourself down very far or are unable to bring yourself up more than a few times. This can be very discouraging for many people and cause them to give up on it. A tip for beginners is to roll the wheel out towards a wall. This break will help to stop you from becoming over extended and past the point that you can safely return to the starting position. Over time as you become better with the exercise you can move further and further from the wall until you no longer need the safety net. Next up, it can be hard on your lower back. The exercise could cause a strain on your lower back as you will need to fight to keep it stable during the exercise. If you are someone that has back problems then you will need to seriously consider it before trying the product. Finally, like all exercises you need to be able to perform it with good form or you will be risking injury. As you begin the exercise ease into it, focus on keeping your body tight and inline. You will get far more out of doing the exercise properly with good form than with sloppy form. Quality over quantity is always something to remember when exercising.

In the end I find that the Ab Wheel is worth the tiny investment in time and money. You might find that it will provide you with a great workout to add to your daily routine or just something that you can use to break up your current exercises. Just be mindful of the safety concerns associated with the product as well as your own limitation. You might find that the ab wheel will become your most loved and hated piece of workout equipment!

81

Fat Fighters

There are so many products out there that claim to be the secret to success and provide you with a short cut. Often these miracle short cuts come in the form of a pill that you take before or after a meal. One such pill is known as fat fighters or blockers. The claim is simple, take the pill around the time you eat something and it will help to prevent you from absorbing all of the calories, fats, or carbs. That sounds like such a great product doesn't it! Eat all you want and just take the pill and your body won't absorb as much of the things that can lead to poor health and weight gain. Sound too good to be true?

One of the major problems in the supplement world is that supplements are not regulated by the FDA (Food and Drug Administration). What does that mean? Well, it means that a company doesn't have to follow the guidelines other products have to follow. This often times leads to exaggerated or false claims, and incomplete ingredient lists. So you might not even know what is in the supplement that you are taking! Think about that for a moment, we have been focusing on monitoring what we put in our bodies for almost 3 months now and if you are taking something like a fat fighter you might not know what is even in it. A good example of how this could be a major problem is that some popular brands have ingredients that are being looked at for their potential blood sugar lowering properties. So for a diabetic this could conflict with their medications leading to an inability to balance their blood sugar level. We have gone over the dangers of that earlier so I won't spend any time on it now.

So far there has been no research done that shows that the pills are able to do what they claim. So the claim that you can just take a pill and all of your dietary concerns will be gone is just simply not supported by science. What is true about the product is the very real side effects that many experience. To name a few, increased hunger, tiredness, nausea, bloating, gas, diarrhea, menstrual bleeding, and low blood sugar. My personal opinion on it is that the people taking the pills are doing nothing but paying 30 or more dollars for a pill to make them feel bad and use the bathroom more.

Your best bet is to save your money and wellbeing and avoid the miracle pills you see your old friends from high school you haven't talked to in years hawking on social media. Your doctor might prescribe you medication to aid you in your weight loss and you should always consult your doctor before beginning any medication. For the most part though, there are no short cuts. Continue to follow calorie and portion control, and you will see results that are sustainable over the long term. Remember this is a life style change to not only change your body composition through weight loss but to also set you on a path to live a healthier life with reduced risk of chronic preventable illness.

82

Apple Cider Vinegar

Let's continue with another miracle weight loss remedy that you have more than likely have been exposed to. That is the various apple cider vinegar drinks and concoctions that we have all seen and heard about. I am not going to focus on any one single type of apple cider vinegar remedy since there are so many versions out there. Instead we are going to look at the apple cider vinegar itself and decide if there are any weight loss properties it might hold.

First we are going to learn what it is. Apple cider vinegar, or ACV for short is what you get when you take apples and crush the juice out of them. Yeast and bacteria's are then added to the apple juice to cause chemical changes and boom you have apple cider vinegar. It should be noted this process is not unique to apple cider vinegar. Now what are some of the claims with the different concoctions and uses around the product? The first one and most obvious is weight loss, some of the others include appetite suppression and reduction in blood sugar levels. What does the science say thought?

First up with the weight loss there has not been a great deal of research done on the concept yet. One study took 175 obese people and put them on a 12 week plan. There were 3 groups, group 1 had a placebo, and group two took 1 table spoon of ACV while the 3rd group consumed 2 table spoons of ACV. The results showed that after 12 weeks there was a difference in weight loss, but even in the group receiving the higher dose of ACV there was only an average loss of a little over 4 pounds. So does the weight loss idea of apple cider vinegar have some life in it? There is a problem; first the weight loss is so slight that it is almost negligible. Furthermore the study relied on self-reporting dietary journals, and as we know people are really bad at properly recording their food intake. Self-reporting is often considered the most unreliable method in the research field.

Up next is the idea that it is an appetite suppressant. There is a little bit of research that shows that this could also be a possibility, however the researchers concluded that although the subjects did not feel as hungry after taking the ACV it was most likely due to them feeling nauseous. These findings also support the idea behind the results of first study we went over. The participants might have shown weight loss due to them feeling to nauseous to eat! Something that we do know is that there does appear to be blood sugar lowering properties but this is not exclusive to apple cider vinegar and is more of a property of vinegar in and of itself. It should also be noted that the blood sugar lowering brought on by the vinegar seems to be most effective when it is being consumed by someone who is already diabetic.

So what is the verdict? Well, I would say that for now it is not something that you can use to aid in your weight loss. The one study we covered showed that participants who took it did lose weight, albeit a small amount over 12 weeks. The other research showed that people did not eat as much because they were feeling nauseous. When you combine the two you very well might find the reason for the weight loss present in the first study. Now is a time to take a moment and think it through. If the participants lost weight because they were feeling too nauseous to eat then in the end it boils down to the participants likely reduced the total amount of calories that they were eating during the day leading them to the weight loss. Calories in vs calories out would be at play here even if it was not the intentions of the participants. It would seem that taking the ACV really wont aid in your weight loss unless you think that feeling sick will prevent you from eating. There also doesn't seem to be any benefits to apple cider vinegar over any other type of vinegar. In fact any nutritional benefits that you might get from ACV would likely be greater from just eating a regular apple.

Next time you see or hear the wonders of ACV and its effects on weight loss just remember any likely benefit is only to force you to feel too sick to eat. Which in turn is only supporting the idea that weight loss all comes down to calories in vs calories out. I think by now you are realizing that it is a lot easier for you to replace a high calorie food with a low calorie food to reduce your calorie intake than it would be to drink ACV and feel too sick to eat.

83

Body Types

This can be a complicated topic, but I am going to do my best to break it down for you over the next few sections. Have you ever heard the claim that "It's just my body type" when it comes to reasons for weight gain or lack of weight loss? Chances are that you have heard this statement in some variation or another. The chances are that they are referring to being one of the 3 commonly used classifications for body types. Ectomorph, Endomorph, and finally Mesomorph are the classifications we will be going over. Is there any evidence to back it up?

You might be surprised to find out that these classifications date back all the way to the 1940's! They were originally created by Dr. William H. Sheldon when he conducted a study on thousands of university students. Dr. Sheldon classified the participants on a scale of 1 to 7 and placed them into one of the three body types I mentioned earlier. He did not take into account any factors such as diet or exercise routines when classifying the bodies. He thought that he would be able to make a connection between body types and other traits such as intelligence, personality and even morality. In the end the research has been widely discredited, and it appears that his work was based off of the pseudoscience of eugenics that was popular at the time. Still thought the 3 types of body classifications stuck, mostly because it is a convenient way to describe body types in day to day life as well as within the science community.

There is some evidence to show that your body type could help to predict your abilities in things like sports.

However one of the main problems with the 3 body type classification is the idea that you are born into your body type and that is how it is going to be. The truth is that there is a lot of grey area here, and some of what we have already learned can be applied to disproving the notion. Some of us appear to respond better or faster to muscle building exercises and the same can be said for weight loss. On the weight loss side we know that there are a lot of factors at play and the principle of NEAT can make a huge difference in a persons perceived ability or inability to lose weight. In the realm of muscle gain everyone is different. Some people might gain in muscle size with resistance training while others do not. Things like Golgi tendons which help regulate the stretch and contraction of muscles could cause someone's muscles to be able to exert more force than someone who has larger muscles.

Don't fall into the belief that you are born into your body type and there is no way out of it. There are factors you cannot change like bone structure, but you are in control of your weight and muscle. If you want to lose weight increase your activity and decrease your calorie intake. If you want to gain muscle or endurance, train your muscles through resistance. It is up to you to create the body that you want.

84

Body Types: Ectomorphs

Although the idea of being stuck in your body type classification is not exactly true as I mention it can still be a useful method for classifying a person's body. As we have gone over before I believe that it is important for you to have as much knowledge as possible to make good informed health decisions going forward. With that in mind we are going to go over each of the 3 different body types starting with Ectomorphs.

Ectomorphs are classified as being long and lean. They have very little body fat and usually do not have a large amount of muscle mass. Often time's people in this category are accused of being naturally skinny. One of the downfalls associated with the ectomorph body type is an inability to gain muscle. For men they might hate this because they could see it as a natural blocker to them being able to get big muscles. On the women's side of the fence, they might feel that they will never be able to get the "curves".

If you find yourself in this category remember you are not trapped here. Yes it might feel like you are the hard gainers when it comes to the gym but again there is likely more at play here than meets the eye. If you want to gain muscle you need two things. Resistance training to force your muscles to grow and enough calories consumed to help your body build the muscle. Remember back in the NEAT section. Naturally skinny people are more than likely just more active than the average person is. If an ectomorph is having trouble putting on weight, be it fat or muscle the truth is that they are just not eating enough. Increasing your resistance training through progressive overload, increasing the weight of the resistance as you get stronger, and increasing your calorie consumption you will see results. You might think you are eating a lot of food, and you very likely could be. However are you eating enough to overcome the energy you burn through exercise and NEAT?

85

Body Types: Endomorphs & Mesomorphs

The other two classification types are Endomorphs and Mesomorphs. It is likely that if you are reading this book you fall into the endomorph classification, and you might not have liked the prior section on ectomorphs and their problems not consuming enough food. You might find this section more to your liking.

To start we are going to cover mesomorphs. People in this classification are muscular and well built. They are the ones that you see in the gym with the big muscles and the relatively low body fat percentage. Most people in the category have to work to get there; it might be through hours spent in the gym or through a physical labor job. The point is that they have kept their diets in check and provided their muscles with enough resistance overtime to force muscle growth. It is likely that they have an elevated metabolism due to their exercise or work habits and their large muscle mass. Usually when someone in this category stops exercising or training their muscles they will lose their muscle mass or gain fat, supporting the idea that you can move in between body types.

Next we have endomorphs, your likely starting category. People in this category are usually big with a high percent of body fat. There is little to no muscular definition that can be seen due to the high level of body fat over the muscles. An endomorph could have a large amount of muscle mass under their layer of body fat but it is also just as likely they have low levels of muscle mass. You might see some professional athletes such as football linemen fall into this category. It is possible for a person in this category to lose body fat and enter into either of the other two categories through adjustments to diet and exercise routines. Again supporting the fact that you are not stuck in any one body classification category.

It is common for people to fall back on the thought that their body classification is set and they are just living with it. The fact is that you can move in an out of each category, the problem is that it is usually hard work. If an endomorph wants to be a mesomorph then they need to reduce their calorie intake to lose weight and increase their resistance training to increase muscle. It is not easy but it is something that attainable. If an endomorph wants to be an ectomorph then again reducing calorie intake to lose body fat is what is needed to be done. It is your body, and your choices shape it. The body classification system has been an excuse for millions of people don't let it be yours.

Negative Calorie Foods.

This is an interesting concept that I have both heard and been questioned about often. The basic idea is that there are foods out there that you can eat that take more calories to chew and digest than what you get from the actual food. In short you burn more by eating them then you gain. Think for a moment have you heard this before, what is the food that has been in the back of your mind since you read the title of the section. I am going to take a wild guess here and say you have been thinking about celery. Was I right?

This concept also goes by the name 0 calorie foods. I already mentioned one of the ones that I hear about most often. Some of the other ones I have seen are apples, beets, garlic, grapefruit, cauliflower, and carrots. The list goes on and on, but did you notice something about the short list I provided, or the ones that you might have heard of and I didn't mention? They are all fruits and vegetables. The only foods that are out there that have no calories are water, and foods we engineered such as diet sodas. Foods with no calories just do not exist, but that is not what the claim was now is it? The claim is that there are foods out there that are so low in calories that you burn more digesting them than you absorb from them. Well time to be the barer of bad news, those foods do not exist either.

Yes there are foods out there with really low calorie counts; we have gone over a handful of them in previous sections. However there are no foods out there that cost more energy than they provide. We know that a calorie is a calorie, but we also know that a calorie is made up from the proteins, carbohydrates and fats found in the foods we eat. Furthermore you know that nutrients are broken down and consumed at different rates depending on their chemical makeup. Some nutrients take more energy to breakdown than others. This means that part of the idea of negative calorie foods is sort of correct. Some foods will cost more energy to be broken down and digested than other. Fats typically take the least amount of energy in the digestion process, usually costing about 3 percent of what is consumed. For fibrous fruits and vegetables you are going to burn about 20 percent of the calorie intake on digestion. For your proteins you are looking at up to 30 percent of the calories consumed to be used to digest the food.

Looking at that math there are ways you can set yourself up for success when it comes to burning calories in digestion. However there is no way for you to burn more than you consume when we are talking about just the digestive process alone. I always like to note that you should not try to factor in the calories burnt from digestion when counting your calories for the day. One it adds another level of record keeping and two it might cause you to consume more calories during the day. When you are counting your calories always air on the side of caution. Follow what the calorie count is on the labels or nutritional information, this will ensure that you are able to stay within your calorie range. When you break it all down to far you are opening up a higher risk for error, and when you have errors in your calorie count you will only be slowing your progress.

The final point I would like to make about the negative calorie foods is that just because the concept is not true that doesn't mean you shouldn't "try it". By that I mean that the foods that fall into that category are both low in calories and high in fiber. Go ahead and think about what he have already learned! Fiber can greatly aid our digestive system. It can help to reduce digestive issues as well as slow down digestion making us feel fuller longer. Adding the low calorie high fiber foods into your diet can help to keep you from consuming other foods with higher calorie counts throughout the day. If you haven't already introduced more plant based foods into your daily diet it might be time for you to consider it. It might just be the boost that you need!

87

As Seen on TV: Slender tone belts

With the early focus of this book being on dietary changes you might have noticed some of the focus has switched to other areas of the health and fitness world. The truth is that you should still be monitoring your calorie intake and portion control; there are only so many sections I can cover on that. It is important for everyone to know how to navigate the diet industry and other health concepts if you want to make the changes you have made permeant. Going over a variety of health and nutritional claims, as well as, products out there shows you how to spot the good from the bad. Remember you are working towards a lifestyle change and with that comes a well-rounded knowledge on what you need to do to get yourself into a healthy state and how to keep yourself there. Let's continue with a review of another popular as seen on TV product, which promotes a short cut to fitness. The slender tone electrical belts.

I still see new versions of this product pop up on my TV from time to time. What the product usually advertises is a device (usually a belt) that you put on your body and it provides an electrical pulse to your muscles. This pulse will cause your muscles to contract and release, very similar to if you were exercising that muscle group. The advertisement typically shows someone with well defined muscles such as a six pack, and it shows them doing the exercise while watching TV or at the office. Is your quackery alarm going off in your head yet? It should be. In this description you are seeing a couple things, first a short cut to being fit. Secondly, unrealistic results from the product. Let's take a look at some of the research just to be sure though.

The concept seems sound, the electrical pulse causes a muscle contraction which then leads to muscle growth. It is not that simple, muscles grow to respond to the resistance placed on them. This is why are you become stronger with resistance training you need to gradually keep adding more and more resistance to the exercise if you want your body to respond by increasing muscle. When the muscle contraction is caused by the electrical pulse there is no resistance, so no real muscle growth is going to take place. Additionally since the contraction is being conducted by the electrical impulse you are not going to burn energy in the process of the contraction. In the end you won't be building any muscle, and you won't be burning any additional calories so what is the point? There is still a use for the electrical stimulation devices, but it is more in the realm of muscle recovery that anything else. Although, you should leave that up to the medical professionals.

All in all the product will be a big waste of your time and money. Stick to perfecting your diet and increasing your activity level if you want to see results.

88

Calorie Tip: Cauliflower

This is will be a short section, but one that might lead you to an alternative food source that could make a big impact on your life. The cauliflower isn't usually the first thing that people grab when (if) they are craving a vegetable, but is one that you might be surprised to find out is very versatile. That's right the little white broccoli looking vegetable could be the key to reducing the calorie content of some of your favorite foods!

Ok that last part might not be all that correct but it gets you in the mind set for what is being covered in this section. We are inching our way toward the end of our third month! With that you have probably been out there doing some of your own research looking for healthy food alternatives. You may or may not have come across the many uses of the cauliflower in your research. It has become popular in the past few years as a means of replacing aspects of your favorite foods, making them have fewer calories and better nutrients. First let's look at some of the nutritional information for cauliflower. A whole head of the stuff contains 146 calories, that's a lot of food for very little calorie content! It is low in fat and carbs but high in protein, potassium, and a variety of vitamins and minerals. It will also provide you with a large amount of fiber.

Now here is where your own research is going to come into play. I would love to write several pages on the foods you can replace with cauliflower but that is not what this book is. Instead I will cover a few of the things I have seen it used in place of. One of my favorites is hot wings. Now I am not saying that it is a perfect replacement for the spicy chicken wing, however it is a great alternative. With a little prep and baking time you can create a hot wing style snack that taste great with a fraction of the calories and fat as the real thing. Next up mash potatoes. Some people have found that with the proper prep you can create a mash potato alternative with half the calories. Finally I have seen pizza crust be replaced with cauliflower. Many people love pizza, but with that love comes a high calorie and high carb bill. Replacing the doughy pizza crust with a low calorie alternative might allow you to enjoy your pizza without the big hit to your daily calorie allowance.

     I provided just a few quick examples of ways that you are able to use cauliflower to replace or alter some of your favorite foods to provide a lower calorie alternative. If this is something that you are interested in, I suggest that you do a little bit of research on your own and find some recipes you might enjoy. You might surprise yourself with how many different ways you can make small adjustment's to your favorite foods to reduce their calorie content!

89

Alcohol

Don't freak out, I do not have any plans to ruin the occasional drink for you like I might have ruined soda and fruit juices. Ok, well it might still happen. Not everyone reading this book is a drinker, some of you might be while other are not. The point of this section is to just give a brief review of some information on nutrition, and to provide my own interpretation of the data.

Starting with nutrition, it is likely that if you have been reading your food labels and keeping track of your calories then if you have consumed an alcoholic beverage you probably have looked at the nutrition label. What did you see there? Well that depends on what you were drinking. For a beer it could have been anywhere from 55 calories up to almost 300 calories! This is because there are so many different types and brands out there. There is a section of the beer market that is created for people conscious of their calorie intake, these come in the forms of light beers and usually weigh in under 150 calories. There are also many options with under 100 calories. Once you start to get into your regular beers and lagers you will see a big spike in the number of calories. The pattern seems to follow the heavier the beer the more calories there will be. What about if you were to drink wine?

Wine can be a little deceiving for a couple of reasons. First, like beer there are many many different types of wine and with that comes a large variety of ingredients. Secondly a serving size of wine is typically only 5oz; that is less than half the typical serving size of beer. Depending on your glass it could be very easy to consume well over the 5 ounces in a serving and not even notice. With the typical calorie count for a serving of wine being around 125 calories, over consuming could really add up the calories quickly! One of the other issues with wine can be the sugar amounts. The average red or white wine will usually contain around 1 gram of sugar. However there are others that can contain 7 grams or more per-serving!

As I mentioned earlier, if you have been watching your calories and eating the correct portion sizes then the amount of calories in alcoholic beverages should not come as a surprise to you. I know for many of the people reading this book you might enjoy the occasional drink or night out. In all honesty that is completely fine, but if you are serious about your weight management and reaching or maintain your goal weight then you do a little prep beforehand. Start including a night out in your calorie plan for the day, this will ensure that you know how many calories you can consume that night and not go over your daily allowance. Next research the nutritional facts about the drinks that you drink or plan to drink. Look for the low calorie beverages, there are many to choose from. Finally stay within your calorie range for the day. One night out of over consumption could set you back further than you ever thought!

90

Reflection

Today is the 90th day since you started this book, not only is it the half way point for the sections of this book; it is also a huge mile stone! Today we are not going to focus on learning anything new, instead I want you to dedicate this day to self-reflection. We are at 3 months in now, and that is a bigger accomplishment then what you might have thought it was! I want you to take a moment and think on a few things

News reports show that the average person gives up on a diet at about 5 weeks. We are sitting at around 12 weeks today! Think back on other restrictive diets you have tried in the past, does that 5 week quitting point sound about right? You might not have completely given up on your diet at that point, but did you start to falter a little? Lose motivation? Begin to cheat more and more? How do you feel this time around? By now many of the new life style habits you have been implementing should start to become part of your daily routine without much thought. Are you beginning to find the methods in this book to be easier to maintain than restrictive diets you have tried in the past?

Take today and really reflect on the choices that you have made up to this point. Are you taking the steps needed to accurately record your daily calorie intake? Are you taking the time to control your portion sizes? Do you opt for the lower calorie options now? Finally, the most important question you need to ask yourself. Are you 100% committed to making the necessary life style changes you need to live a healthier life? Are you able to do more? Think hard on this, can you do more in this journey? That means can you do more to control your nutrition, and can you do more to improve your activity levels?

At this point in your journey, if you have been sticking to your caloric needs and maintaining a 15-25 percent calorie deficit daily then you should have seen positive results by now. If you have not then it is time for you to go back to the drawing board and reassess your TDEE, calorie intake, portion sizes, and activity level. For the next 30 days we are going to be focusing on your physical fitness and maintaining your calorie deficit. I hope that you have been taking your physical activity seriously because in the next section we are going to go over some information that will help you to take it to the next level! You might not be ready to do some of the things that we are going to be covering over the next month but keep reading because one day this will be useful to you!

91

Reassess Your TDEE

As I stated in the last section if you have been fully committed to controlling your energy intake and output then by this point you should have seen some results. Some of you might have seen tremendous results while for others the progress might have been slower. Remember this is a marathon not a sprint, you should not be expecting to lose 40 or more pounds in the first 3 months. However since it has been 90 days it could be time for you to recheck your TDEE.

Remember that TDEE stands for total daily energy expenditure; it is the amount of calories that you are expected to burn based on your current weight and activity level. If you have lost weight then your body will need fewer calories then when you started. Reassessing your TDEE will allow you to keep an accurate estimate of how manty calories you need at your lighter weight. Take the time now to reassess your TDEE:

First you need to find your BMR (basal metabolic rate):

- Men: BMR = 66 + (6.23 X weight in pounds) + (12.7 X height in inches) – (6.8 X age)
- Women: BMR = 655 + (4.35 X weight in pounds) + (4.7 X height in inches) – (4.7 X age)

Next multiply your BMR number by your activity TDEE number:

Sedentary: Little to no exercise, desk job, most of the day spent sitting or not moving much

- TDEE = 1.2xBMR

Lightly Active: Very light exercise; make a small effort to not be sitting all day.

- TDEE = 1.375xBMR

Moderately active: You make an effort to be active, might hit the gym a little or go for walks often

- TDEE= 1.55xBMR

Very Active: You exercise heavily every day, you might have a very physical job, you make your fitness a priority in your life.

- TDEE = 1.725xBMR

Extremely active: Very heavy exercise routine/physical job. Likely an athlete or you exercise several times a day.

- TDEE = 1.9xBMR

If your goal is still to lose weight I recommend that you select an activity level for your TDEE formula that is lower than your actual activity level. Doing this will lower your TDEE calorie count and aid you in maintaining a calorie deficit. When you estimate your TDEE activity level to high then it is possible you will believe you are burning more calories than you are. This will affect your daily calorie deficit and could slow your progress. It boils down to this; if you believe your TDEE is 2,200 calories a day based on your activity level but your actual TDEE level is 2,000 calories a day then you might be reducing your calorie deficit by 200 calories a day. Over the course of the week that's 1,400 calories and in a single month that reaches 6,000 calories you didn't need to eat. Slowing your progress by almost 2 pounds in a month, all from over estimating your TDEE level.

Now that you know your new TDEE number you can create a new daily calorie deficit goal. Remember to aim for a goal of cutting your TDEE by 15-25 percent per day. It is important that you do not cut too much out or you risk becoming malnourished. On the other side if you do not cut out enough then you will not see results. It is important to find a balance that works for you. Continue to closely monitor your portion control and make sure you are achieving your daily nutritional needs!

92

Gym Fear

For many people going to the gym is a scary thought. There is equipment I don't know how to use. I can barely even do push-up. People will judge me. I need to get in better shape at home before I try to go to a gym. Do any of those excuses ring a bell for you? For many people working up the courage to go to the gym is an impossible task. Don't worry this section is not going to play out the way you might think.

I am not going to tell you that it's *all* in your head and that people really don't care that an out of shape or bigger person is in the gym. The truth is that if you go to the gym as an overweight person you are going to get judged and stared at. If you go to the gym as an underweight you are going to get stared at. If you go to the gym as an average person you are going to get judged and stared at. Are you picking up the pattern here? The gym can be a very harsh judgmental place, but it can also be a fantastic place to meet new people and achieve your fitness and weight loss goals.

The thing that you need to understand about going to the gym is that it is not unlike other public places you go to. There are people going about their business doing what they went there to do, the same as someone going out to do their grocery shopping. Some people are nice, some people are rude, and there are people who fall everywhere in between. The gym is no different, it is made up of a variety of people who could be rude to you, could be helpful to you, or might just ignore you. We are going to take a moment and go over some of the things that you might experience when you go to a gym and the possible reasons why this happens.

First, every gym regular sees the gym as "their" gym; it becomes a second home so to speak for many people. It is a place where they have spent hours of their time, built up a reputation and relationships. When someone new enters their "home" they might be skeptical of that person until they show a commitment to the gym. Gym regulars see a lot of people come and go throughout the years, and there is typically a pattern of behavior. A good example is the start of a new year. Gym regulars dread the first 2-3 weeks after the first of the year. The gym becomes crowded with all sorts of people who made their goal to lose weight and get in shape. Over the course of a couple of weeks the crowd will thin out a little more every day until it is back to the regulars plus a couple of people that remained committed to their new year's resolution. This pattern of new people joining the gym; staying for a few weeks then leaving for ever is on repeat during the course of a year. Gym regulars tend to see new people as "in the way" because they see new people as being temporary to the gym, and as such wasting every ones time. Is this a good attitude to have? No, and I am not excusing how new people are treated in the gym. Remember this is not meant to be a feel good book, you are here to learn how things are; not how we would like them to be. New people at the gym can be treated with skepticism at first, it is unfortunate but that's how it often is. Would more new people stick it out longer if they felt more welcomed? Probably, but I don't see this changing any time soon.

People are going to stare at you. This is something that you will just have to get over and realize that it is not exclusive to your weight or fitness level. Everyone gets stared at in the gym. The guy trying to squat 3 hundred pounds as his warm up will get stared at, the high school kid who looks like he is made out of pipe cleaners benching 185 is getting stared at.

The girl who spends more time taking selfies to post on her social media then working out gets stared at. The new out of shape person gets stared at. Not all staring means judgment or disapproval, to be honest it is mostly just curiosity. People want to see if you are actually able to lift that weight; if you are going to do it with good form; if you are going to push yourself or just drop the weight the second you get a little tired. People are curious as to what workout other people are doing, is it a PPL? SL 5x5? Upper lower split? A bro-split? Or a random set of exercises without a reason? Will there be someone staring at you because of your weight? Yes, hate to say it but some people are just not nice.

People are going to make comments both good and bad, as well as give unsolicited advice. People make comments about the overweight person, they make comments about the meat heads, and they make comments about the skinny kid. Not everyone seems to go by the rule of if you don't have something nice to say don't say anything at all, just a fact of life. You might also encounter the "positive" comments about being the big person at the gym. The "good for you" comments are something you will more than likely encounter. Sometimes people feel the need to encourage the overweight person. You can chose to take it as a complement that you are trying to make an active change in your life or you can see it as a negative condescending comment, it is up to you. Finally, you will also get advice from all types of people at the gym. This will range anywhere from diet advice to what workout you should be doing. Sometimes this advice will be correct and often it will be incorrect. The best thing you can do is do your own research and take advice you get with a grain of salt until you can research it yourself. Just because the fit person at the gym gives you advice, that doesn't mean it is correct.

Ok so we have gone over all of the negatives of going to the gym and why you might fear going. The truth is that you might have a bad experience at the gym from time to time, but for most of the time you will be able to go in, do your workout, and go home. No one will care that you are there. It can also be a great way place to meet new people and build relationships with others who share similar goals as you. Surrounding yourself with people who share your goals can be a great way to keep you on track for achieving yours.

The truth is that *most* of your fears of the gym are going to be in your own head. Gyms are really a great place where you can focus on improving your fitness and achieving weight loss goals. If you put in the work you will see results. However you need to make sure that you pick the right gym for you. There are all sorts of options out there when you are considering you gym options. Some cater to power lifter, while other are designed for people who want a workout but not designed for the heavy lifters. It is important that you pick a gym that matches your needs. If you are going to run on a treadmill or use the elliptical then a powerlifting or cross fit style gym won't be for you. If you are trying to pack on muscle with heavy Olympic lifts then Planet fitness probably won't be for you. Research what type of workout you think would be right for you then research your local gyms to pick the one that fits your needs. Many will allow you to use a trial membership so you can get a feel for it before you make a commitment.

Gyms are not terrible places, but there are things that you might have to put up with when you go to one. The important thing is to remember why you are there. You are trying to make a positive change in your life. Stay committed and understand that there will be those who make rude comments, and think you don't belong there. It is a sad fact; don't let it get to you. Stay committed, stay motivated, and do your research.

93

RPE: Rate of Perceived Exertion

As I am sure you have come to notice, not all exercises are created equal. Some exercises require more effort on your part to complete, for example swimming laps in a pool is more taxing on your body than walking a lap around the track. However is the type of exercise the main difference? Or is there something else that influences our exercise results.

The truth is that when it comes to exercise we get out of it what we put into it. In our previous example, swimming laps in a pool can be a very hard exercise; far more difficult than walking. However if the person who is walking laps is really pushing themselves to a point that they are able to get their heart rate elevated for an extended period of time, and the person who is swimming laps is doing so using resting strokes and not pushing themselves then who is going to get more out of their workout? Just doing a "harder" workout does not mean that you will get better results than someone who is doing an "easy" workout. The thing that really matters is how much effort you are putting into your exercise. This is where the RPE: Rate of Perceived Exertion comes into play. The RPE is a method for determining how hard you're exerting yourself during exercise. Because it is a self-assessment it is a great way for you to personalize it to your fitness level. There are two different scales used one runs from 6-20 and the other runs from 1-10. We are going to focus on the scale that runs 1-10 only because I find it to be easier for those who are new to fitness. How it works is simple 1 means the activity is very easy, or no activity at all. 10 is your absolute limit, there is no way you could go harder. The scale is as follows.

1: Very easy, no activity. This is you at rest.

2: Fairly light. This is where you should feel when you are warming up or cooling down. Not Hard.

3: Light exertion: You are moving but it is not difficult. You can easily hold a conversation while at this level.

4: Moderately easy: You are moving now and starting to sweat. You can still hold a conversation at this point, but your breathing and heart rate has increased.

5. Moderate to kind of difficult: You are moving really well now, you are breathing heavy and your heart rate is elevated. Holding a conversation at this point is becoming difficult.

6. Hard: You are working hard now, you cannot hold a conversation but you can speak a few words at a time.

7. Hard to a little intense: Your heart is pounding and your breathing is very heavy. You might be having a hard time maintaining this for long periods of time.

8. Intense: You are breathing very heavy and are getting close to your limits. You can no longer speak without having to gasp for air.

9. Very intense: You are struggling to breath, and unable to keep this pace up for more than a minute or two. Speaking is impossible.

10. Maximum: This is your limit; you will not be able to hold this level for more than 15 to 20 seconds.

As you can see the scale is very easy to follow. Your ability to hold a conversation is a great way to measure your exertion level; the harder it is to speak the harder you are working. Now we know what the RPE is and how the scale works, but how do we apply it? How you use it will depend on your goals. If your goal is to get into better cardiovascular shape then you need to aim to stay in a range around 6 or 7 for 20 to 30 minutes at a time. If your goal is to just move for the sake of getting in more movements, possibly for weight loss, then aiming for a 4-5 would be ideal. For the average person reading this book maintaining an activity in the 4-6 range will be perfect, you are not pushing yourself to your absolute limits but you are working yourself hard enough to burn calories and get your heartrate into an elevated level.

When you are using the scale there are a few things that you need to remember. First, as I said the scale can be applied to your specific fitness level. An activity that might be a 7 for you could be a 4 for someone else because their fitness level might be higher than yours. The second thing you need to remember is that the scale changes for you over time. As you become more fit the activity or pace you use to use to get yourself to reach a level 6 might not be able to get you to that level anymore. After a few months of exercising your level 6 at the beginning might shift down to a level 3. As you become more fit things become easier for you, so in turn as things become easier you need to up your pace or intensity to maintain in the higher levels on the RPE scale.

Give it a try during your next activity. Complete the activity then review the scale and see where you believe you landed. Was it a 2? How about a 5? Once you have figured out where your current activity lands make adjustments to it so that you will be able to get into the desired RPE level. Use the scale as a way to make sure that you are completing each activity or exercise in the proper range. When you are able to remain consistent with the level of exertion in your workouts then you will be able to be consistent with your calorie burned estimations. The more accurate your estimations the better results you will have!

Exercise Vocabulary

With the focus of this month being on exercise we will need to increase your understanding of a few vocabulary terms. Remember the more vocabulary you understand the easier it will be to conduct your own research and develop plans passed this book. The focus of this section will be on the terms surrounding lifting weights and other exercises.

Up first let's cover the term repetition. The simple dictionary definition is the "recurrence of an action or event". In the world of fitness a repetition is how many times you repeat the same action. Let's take the simple bicep curl for an example, when you perform the bicep curl you are lifting a weight in your hand by bending at the elbow and bringing your hand towards your shoulder. The action of lifting the weight from the bottom to the top and back down to the bottom is 1 repetition, or 1 rep for short. That is easy enough! Next up is the term "set" or "sets". You will see the term set go hand in hand with the term repetition. A set is a group of consecutive repetitions. When we are talking about sets it is how many times we will complete the group of repetitions. For example if you are doing 10 repetitions of bicep curls you might be doing 3 sets. This means that you will do the group of 10 bicep repetitions 3 times. In the end you will be completing a total of 30 bicep repetitions in 3 different groups or sets of 10. It can be common for some plans to also include the term "rep range". This term is used to give you a low number and a high number to complete for reps. For example, you might have an exercise that gives you a rep range of 8-10 reps per set. So you should strive to complete a number of repetitions in the range from 8-

10. Once you are able to reach the max for the rep range for all of your sets then it is time to either increase your rep range or increase your resistance in order to keep making improvements.

The next 3 vocabulary terms we will be going over are specific to the action of moving your muscles against a resistance. The first one is the concentric portion of a movement. This is what most people would consider the "contraction" part of a movement. It is when you are tightening or shortening the muscle. Continuing with the same bicep curl example, the concentric phase would be as you lift the weight up. Once you have reached the peak of the exercise, or when your muscle is fully contracted you are now in the isometric contraction. Isometric contractions are pretty simple to understand, it is when a muscle is contracting, although it does not have to be a full contraction, and the angle and movement of the muscle does not change. A good example of this is if you stand in a doorway and press with your arms out against the door frame hard for a minute or two then release. You will be able to feel that your muscles were working but no movement really took place. So simply put an isometric contraction is when you are pulling or pushing against a force but no moment takes place. The final vocabulary term we will talk about is the eccentric contraction. If concentric is the shortening of the muscle, and isometric is the holding of a muscle against resistance, then that really only leaves one other option. The eccentric phase is lengthening of a muscle, or the lowering of the weight. This is part of the exercise when you are lowering the weight back down to the starting position. It is often the most ignored portion of an exercise but it is one of the most important parts. It is important to muscle development, the mind muscle connection, and injury prevention. You need to focus on performing the eccentric portion of an exercise in a slow controlled motion. Lowering too fast or dropping the weight could increase your risk of injury through strain, tears, or hyper extension. It is also part of the muscle building process, so focusing on the eccentric portion of a lifting exercise as much as the other phases gives you extra work in that exercise. Extra work means better results and more calories burnt! If you are going to do something you might as well do it right!

Mind Muscle Connection

If you recall a while back I mentioned the mind muscle connect, and that we would cover it in more detail later in the book. While it is now later in the book, so let's dive right in. The mind muscle connection might sound like a dumb concept on its surface. You might be thinking to yourself, "of course I have the mind muscle connection, my muscles move when my mind tells them to!" You would be kind of correct, but there is more to it than that.

When we talk about the mind muscle connection we are talking about a very specific process that applies to exercise and muscle control. When we talk about the Mind Muscle Connection, MMC for short, we are talking about a very deliberate and conscious effort to contract a muscle. Sitting here reading this book it might be hard for you to imagine this as something more than what you already do, but when you put it into practice you will realize its importance to improving your fitness and getting the most out of each repetition! EMG research has shown that when you focus on a single muscle group during resistance training, you are able to use more of the muscle fibers for the primary movers and fewer accessory muscle fibers. What does this mean? Simply put when you really concentrate on what muscle group you are trying to workout then you will be able to use a higher percentage of the muscle fibers for that muscle group. In short, you are being more efficient with each repetition because you will be using more of primary mover and less of the assister muscle groups.

You can give this a try by doing a simple bicep curl. Pick up something to curl; it can be a weight, a resistance band, a jug of milk, anything that can be used as a resistance against your bicep muscle. Now I want you to curl the weight 10 times without thinking about it, just complete 10 repetitions. Next switch the weight to the other arm and complete 10 curls, but this time focus on only using your biceps muscle. Focus on feeling the bicep muscle contract and tighten. Continue to tighten as your curl the weight up, once the weight is at the top of the curl your bicep should be contracted and tightened as much as you can. You should curl the weight up slowly taking around 2-3 seconds to go from the bottom of the movement to the top. Next reverse the movement by slowly lowering the weight back down. This time focus on slowly releasing the tension out of the bicep as you return back to the start. You should have been able to notice the difference between the 2 arms. The arm that you really concentrated on using the bicep muscle should feel like it received the better workout. This is because you were able to recruit a larger number of muscle fibers in the primary mover due to the extra focus on the muscle.

Don't be discouraged if it did not seem to make as big of a difference for you as what I made it sound. Like everything, practice makes perfect. When it comes to the MMC you need to practice it, and the more focus you place on it the better your results will be. As you feel each specific muscle contracting during your exercise you will notice that it will become easier and easier to isolate the different muscle. Think of it as building up more precision in your muscle use, the more you train your mind to focus on which muscle you want to use the more precise your movements will become. This is a skill that you will find is common in high performing athletes. High performance athletes typically will have fantastic hand eye coordination. This is a result of having a great MMC, which allows the athlete to recruit their muscle to perform very specific precise movements.

As the relationship between your mind and your muscles improves you will find that things like your hand eye coordination will improve. You will find that you will be able to isolate specific muscles you want to flex. Much like the body builders on stage who are able to pick out a specific muscle to flex, you will be able to isolate your different muscle groups as well.

Now what is the best way to improve your mind muscle connection? We already went over the best methods, and that is slowing down your exercise. No matter what exercise you are performing you will be able to focus on a specific muscle group that is the primary mover. You need to concentrate on this muscle group for both the concentric and eccentric phase of the exercise. When in the concentric phase you are contracting the muscle, it is important in this phase to not be swinging the weight or using any sort of momentum to aid in lifting the weight or resistance. You might have heard of "cheat curls", which is when you swing the weight to build momentum to help you lift it easier. Not only is this just wasting your time because you are using momentum to lift the weight and not your muscle, you are also not building up the MMC because you are not isolating a specific muscle group in the exercise. Go nice and slow, some research has shown that a repetition should take about 10 seconds to complete. Take 4 seconds to lift the weight up, this is the concentric phase. Hold the weight at the peak or isometric contraction, where your muscle is fully tightened and flexed, for 2 seconds. Then lower the weight in the eccentric phase taking another 4 seconds. This will help you to really focus on isolating the muscles you are trying to work out and give you the best results. Think quality of repetitions over quantity.

During your next work out session give this method a try. It will take some practice to get it right, and it might take a while to get use to slowing down and focusing on a specific muscle. Once you start to notice your MMC you will be surprised out how much more efficient your workouts will become!

DOMS: Delayed Onset Muscle Soreness

If you have ever worked out or did some physical activity beyond what you usually do then you likely experienced some muscle soreness in the days following. This is known as delayed onset muscle soreness, DOMS for short. We don't know a great deal about the specific causes of DOMS but what we do know is that it can be very uncomfortable and even down right painful! What can I tell you about it though?

First DOMS can be characterized by pain or soreness in your muscles following an intense activity or an activity that you are not use to. This can be common for people who are new to exercise or if you switch up your standard exercise program. The soreness typically begins within the first two days following the exercise and can last for 24-48 hours. But what is the cause of the soreness? One theory is that it is caused by micro-trauma in the muscles. The popularity of this theory is probably rooted in the idea that when you use your muscles they are broken down and need to rebuild. The idea seems sound, you breakdown muscle and it results in muscle pain while they "heal". However, this is likely not the cause of DOMS. Another possible cause of DOMS could be a form of Rhabdomyolysis, which is a condition where muscle protein is spilled into the blood stream. Of course there are many other theories on what the real culprit is, but the cause really doesn't matter too much.

What I am sure you are really interested in is how to prevent or reduce the effects of DOMS on yourself. There are a few things you might be able to do to reduce your rate of DOMS. First is to just suck it up and get past it. Typically once your body begins to adjust to your new activity level the amount of DOMS that you feel reduces to a point that you won't even notice it anymore. I know that is easier said than done, but the truth is that DOMS is not permanent and it will not happen after every workout. The other thing that you can do to reduce the level of DOMS that you feel is to ease into the workouts.

Easing into your workout is a great way to allow your body to adjust to the new activity and prevent as much soreness. People are often too quick to think that they can just go to the gym and max out in everything only to find out the next morning how sore they are. A few things will often happen as a result. The extreme DOMS that you might experience could cause you to miss several workout sessions, pushing back your progress. It might also cause you to have no desire to return to the same workout because of how sore you became. When you are beginning a new workout routine and want to ease into it, try using the RPE scale that we reviewed in a previous section. Beginning in a range between 2 and 4 will mean that you are getting a workout but you are not going to overdo it. After a few sessions increase your exertion until you are at the level that you want to be at!

97

Lifting Weights as a Woman

Men reading this book, sorry but this section will pertain to the women, now that doesn't mean skip it because it might help you to better inform others. Women, there is a big misconception out there that you are supposed to leave the weights and machines alone and just run on the elliptical and nothing else. The fact is that this couldn't be any further from the truth!

There are many reasons behind the idea that women should avoid the weight room, but the main one I hear most often is the old "I don't want to look buff, or manly". What you need to know is that becoming buff is not some easy thing to do. For women you will have an even harder time becoming "buff" than men do. This is because of the biological differences between men and women. Women have higher levels of estrogen and lower levels of testosterone than their male counter parts. Testosterone is a big player when it comes to muscle development, women naturally have a lower level of it. This means that lifting weights will not make you look like Mr. Olympia.

Ok, so now we know that simply lifting weights is not going to cause women to balloon up, what will lifting weights do for you? First and foremost it will help to build up muscle that will burn more calories throughout the day, so in short it can help to increase your TDEE. Next, you will reshape your body. Exercising your muscles will have a tightening and toning effect for everyone, but for women you might find that it will help you to tighten up some of your trouble areas or the areas you would like to emphasize. Beyond the appearance benefits from weight training there are medical benefits as well. The American Heart Association has approved weight training as beneficial exercise for your health. Research has shown that it can reduce your risk of heart disease! Other medical benefits include bone health. As women age they run a higher risk of developing osteoporosis, research has shown that resistance training can help to increase your bone density. It also appears that the sooner you begin resistance training the better your chance of preventing osteoporosis will be.

If you are looking into what type of exercise you would like to complete consider giving resistance training a try. You might be surprised at just how many benefits you are able to gain by leaving the elliptical and picking up some weights! We will be going over several weight training programs in the coming sections but feel free to do a little research on your own to find the best match for you and your goals!

98

Progressive Overload

Progressive over load is something that you will hear often in the fitness and weight lifting community. Although this section is short, it will be very important for your fitness endeavors going forward! We have gone over a little about what happens to the body when we exercise. Remember exercise is applying a stress to the body, this could come in the form of stress on our cardiovascular system or it could be a stress placed on our muscles through strength training exercises. As a result of the stress our bodies will grow and adapt to match the exercise requirements you are placing on them. This doesn't happen overnight but given proper time, nutrition, and rest our bodies are capable of amazing things. As our bodies adapt to the stresses that we place on them those stresses will become easier. For example running a mile right now might take everything you got, but after a few months running a mile might be your warm up. It is the same for strength training, right now squatting 100 pounds might give you DOMS so bad that you can't sit properly for a week. Given enough time though, a 100 pound squat will be a breeze. This is where Progressive Overload comes into play.

Progressive overload can simply be defined as a gradual increase in stress placed on the body during exercise training. It is very likely that if you have already begun working out to one degree or another then you have naturally implemented progressive overload into your training. Basically what this all boils down to is this. When you are performing an exercise it might be very difficult, and as you keep doing the exercise your body adapts to it and it is no longer as difficult.

Now you are faced with a choice; keep doing the exercise exactly the same and no longer force your body to adapt, or increase something in the workout to force the body to continue to grow and change. In order for your body to continue to grow and change you will need to increase the stress you are placing on it. This is called progressive overload.

This does not happen just over a single workout, progressive overload occurs over months or even years. As an exercise becomes easier you need to slowly increase the stress from that exercise to keep your body adapting. How you progressive overload can be different, and there are many ways that you can accomplish it. If you are strength training you can slowly increase the resistance of the exercise; basically just add more weight to the lifts you are performing. This increase in weight will result in a harder workout for your muscles, and force them to continue to grow. Another method following the same idea is to increase your number of sets or repetitions for that exercise. Increasing frequency of the exercise is another great progressive overload strategy. Going back to our example of lifting weights, if you are exercising a certain muscle group once a week; you can try increasing that workout to twice a week. Other strategies include increasing your RPE, rate of perceived exertion. As well as reducing your rest time between each exercise. If you are running a mile and it is becoming easier and easier, you might need to increase your effort in the exercise to ensure that you are remaining at the RPE level that provides you with an appropriate level of a workout.

Remember that in order for your body to adapt and continue to improve your fitness you will need to increase your workout, or workout intensity. Doing the same exact workout for months on end without any progressive overload will maintain you at whatever fitness level you are at, in short you will "peak" and show no improvement. To properly progressively overload you need to slowly increase, and there are ways that you can check for when you need to increase your workout stress. We have already gone over the two major ones! You can check your workout to your RPE scale and see if you are remaining in your desired range or if the workout is becoming too easy and your level of exertion is dropping. Another great method is to use your "rep ranges". Think back on your vocabulary, a rep range is a numerical range of reps consisting of a low end and a high end. When you increase the load of the workout you should be hitting the low end of the rep range. Overtime you will slowly be able to hit the high end of the rep range. Once you are able to hit your high end of the rep range for all of your sets then it is time to progressive overload! Keep it simple, do not over do it! Increase the stress a little at a time, so for weight training maybe only go up by 5 or less pounds. For endurance training add a little distance, or aim for a faster time by 10 seconds or so. You will be amazed at how quickly your body will adjust and grow when you apply proper training techniques!

High Weight Low Reps VS Low Weight High Reps

I once heard a very true statement about the battle between high reps low weight versus low weight high reps. If you would like to see a fight break out then walk into a gym and say one is better than another. Everyone will have their own opinion on the subject, they will be throwing out research they read, their own experience, and swear by one or the other. This is something that has been a part of the fitness community for decades, but what is the truth? Does one really do better than the other? This section we are going to try to answer those questions. Spoiler! I might make some diehard fans in each group angry.

The conventional wisdom in the gym is that you need to do high weight low reps to build up big muscles and lots of strength and on the other side lifting less weight but for more repetitions you will gain strength but there will be more of a toning effect. Does that sound familiar; have you heard something similar before? As I mentioned, this has been the conventional wisdom for decades, but the research might say something different. Before we get into the research though I would like you to take a moment and think about what we have learned so far and apply it. Think about the RPE scale and how over time your body will adapt, consider the principles of progressive overload. Does that information make you believe that one is better than the other? Are they the same?

The truth is that to a degree both sides are correct, but like many things in the fitness world it is not a simple black and white answer. When you are doing a higher weight lower rep exercise you are performing an anaerobic exercise, so no oxygen is getting used. This could aid in building up strength and size in the muscles, think back to our fitness components sections on muscle strength and muscle endurance. When you are performing an exercise with lower weight but higher reps you will be relying on the aerobic system to fuel your muscles. This could lead to increases in muscle strength as well as muscle endurance. All of that being said, there is a lot of overlap and for the average person it will not make a great deal of difference.

As we mentioned before, our bodies are great at adapting and growing to meet the stress we place on them. If you are lifting weights your muscles are going to grow as long as you are pushing them to. If you are lifting a lower weight for 12 to 15 reps your muscles are still going to improve their strength and grow, unless that weight and 12 to 15 reps become so easy that you are able to perform the exercise with little to no fatigue. The same can be said for a higher weight lower rep range of 3-5 reps. If you are providing adequate stress to the muscles to force them to adapt then they will become bigger and stronger. Some of you might find greater results with one method over the other and that is great for you, but it might not be the same for everyone. The method I prefer to recommend is to try both. We will be covering strength training programs in the coming weeks and some of them will promote the idea of using the both the high weight low rep and the low weight high rep formulas. I recommend using this strategy for people because it will relate back to what we have already learned in our fitness components sections. If you want to have a well-rounded physical fitness level then you need to strive to meet all of the components. If one lifting strategy provides more muscle strength while the other provides more muscle endurance then combining the two will give you a more wholesome fitness level.

If or when you decide to attempt resistance training, try playing around with the low weight high rep and high weight low rep techniques you can tailor them to fit your individual needs and goals. Combining the two strategies is also a great way to keep your routines from becoming stale or boring. It is important to remember that although one might benefit certain aspects in fitness and muscle development more than the other, the amount will vary from person to person and for your level of physical fitness the differences might be too low to worry about at this time. So don't stress out about it!

Oops I Accidently Arnold

This seems to be a good time to go over one of the excuses I hear very often. I call it an excuse because I think that most people who say it know that what they are saying is not true. I am talking about the "I don't want to get to big" line that I often get when I recommend strength training. Have you ever heard this line, or said it yourself?

I have heard the saying "Oops I Accidently Arnold" several times over the years and I like to use it when I hear the excuse of I don't want to get to big. These types of excuses are implying that you can balloon up and look like a body builder (Arnold Schwarzenegger) after only a short period of time in the gym. We all know that to get the muscle size and strength of the body builder types you have to put in long hours at the gym for periods of years, and for some that's not even enough so they turn to steroids and other substances to give them a boost. So it is easy to see why I find this excuse to be so, let's call it annoying and disingenuous. For body builders they put in hundreds of hours at the gym year in and year out focusing on specific muscle development and nutritional needs. For the average person they will never put in the time or the effort needed to reach that size. So it is impossible to "accidently Arnold". You have to be deliberate in your goals and exercise.

For the average person reading this book, if that was one of your concerns then you can put your mind at ease. There is no way that anyone male or female who begin strength training will end up accidently becoming a big blocky muscle head. In fact the results will be very much the opposite. Gaining muscle mass through resistance training will help in the reduction of fat, which as we have learned is about 1.5 times the volume of muscle. Gaining muscle and losing fat will also provide you with a more defined physique often resulting in a slimmer appearance. Yes your muscles will grow some but you won't end up with 17 inch biceps unless you are specifically trying to achieve them!

If you take anything away from this section it is that you need to be deliberate in your plans and activities. Evaluate excuses you might have used or have heard in the past. Are they excuses grounded in reality or are they just excuses used to keep you in the same place in life? Much like the excuse of "I don't want to lift weight because I don't want to get to big", you will find that most excuses are just an excuse to remain the same. We are at 100 days in now and that is a huge accomplishment. I am sure that some of you have already increased your activity level and even developed workouts, others of you might not have yet. If you haven't yet, ask yourself why and be honest! Are your excuses being used to hold you back?

101

Technology

One of the amazing things about living in the time that we do is that there is technology that will aid us in about anything in our lives. We have technology to record our favorite programs automatically; self-driving cars are right around the corner, despite what my grade school teachers claimed I do in fact have a computer/calculator in my pocket most of the day. The world of health and fitness is no different; we have technology that can be used to aid us in counting calories, to counting how many steps we take! Many of you have probably already researched and used some of these technologies in your day to day lives. We are going to take some time to go over a few of them today.

First up we have fitness trackers. The most popular trackers often come in the forms of watches, but many smart phones will have some form of a tracker built right in them. These fitness trackers can be very basic and cheap to very advanced and expensive. Some of the basic functions that are pretty standard are heart rate monitors and step counters. These have shown to be reasonably accurate and are a great way for you to be able to keep track of certain aspects of your physical fitness. We have gone over step trackers previously so I will not take much time on them here, other than to say that having a reminder of how many or few steps you have taken during a day can be a great reminder to either increase your activity or that you are on track. The heart rate monitor can prove to be very beneficial because you can easily track how hard you are working in a given workout based on your heart rate. They can be used to make sure that you are remaining in your target heart rate zone during a cardio workout and not dipping to low.

One of the biggest perceived benefits of fitness trackers is the calorie counting features. This feature works both for calories in and calories out, which sounds like a fantastic tool! A fitness tracker will use your heart rate and step count to give you an estimation on the calories burnt during the day or for a specific workout. While the corresponding software (usually an app on your phone) can track how many calories you eat by plugging what you ate into the app. This is a method for telling how many calories you burnt during the day and how many you consumed. Technology makes that pesky calorie counting so much easier. Does it though? Research has shown that both the calories burnt and consumed can prove to be unreliable with one study showing that the best were off by 27%. Let that number sink in for a moment. Right now you are running at a calorie deficit of 15-25 percent. If you were relying on the calorie counter of a fitness tracker to track your calories in/out then you might still be consuming more than what you need! So if you are planning your meals around the number of calories a device is saying you have burnt or eaten already, then there can be some big problems and you might inadvertently over eat. This is not to say that an activity or fitness tracker wouldn't aid you, but you should not rely on the calorie counters to track your calories consumed and burned. Stick to counting and measuring by hand.

The last bit of technology that I would like to talk about is video games. Not just any video games but those that are interactive with your movements. You know which ones I am talking about; there is the WII, Xbox Kinect, and others. If you are having a hard time finding a workout that you enjoy or gyms are not an option for you at this time consider picking up an interactive gaming system. You can play games that are specifically designed to get you to perform workouts such as dancing games or WII Fit. Or you can try games like Kinect Sports which involves a lot of movement while you compete in entertaining sports games. You might find that adding in 20 minutes of interactive gaming could give you the boost that you need. Now like everything else you will get out of it what you put into it. Don't expect to burn as many calories doing the bowling games as you would playing a full body dancing game.

The important thing is to understand when you are considering using a technology to aid you in your weight loss or physical activity is that you need to select something that you are actually going to use. A step counter isn't going to help you if you do not strive to reach a step goal. A calorie tracker is not going to help you if it is faulty, and finally a gaming system is not going to help you if you hate games or only participate in the ones with minimal activity. You need to select things that fit your needs and goals. Take some time to research what is out there. Maybe there is something that could help you out or fit your needs perfectly. Or maybe you are doing just fine on your own. Make sure that you do your research and more importantly make sure you actually use it or else you are just wasting your money!

102

Is your Fitness Tracker Enough?

In the last section we learned about a few of the technologies out there that people like to use to aid their fitness and weight loss journey. One of the most common ones you see today, and we have spoken about them several times is the fitness trackers. You might have noticed that these little wrist watch styled activity trackers are all over the place. It is likely that many of the people reading this book are currently wearing one. The question though is do they help? We are going to take a look at what some of the research shows us and I'll try to break down that research using the information that we have already covered.

Many people pick up a fitness tracker such as a Fitbit with the idea that it will help them to lose weight. From the reminder of how many steps you have taken today to the alerts it will give you if you have been inactive too long. How can it not help you to lose weight right? This is day 102 so I am sure that you know that if I am asking you questions then the likely result is going to be negative. Well you might be somewhat correct with that one. An activity tracker is fantastic for giving you a reminder that you need to move more, however it will only work if you actually use that reminder to get up and move, and stay consistent with it! When you use the activity tracker as it is intended with a proper diet then you will see the results that you desire. It is when you fail at one or both of those that you will find that you are not going to achieve your goal.

What does the research tell us? There have been several studies done on the effects of fitness trackers and weight loss. The conclusion? Well typically the studies found that those who wear the fitness trackers lose less weight than those who do not. Those results sound a little backwards from what you might expect don't they? How could someone who is having a reminder on their arm telling them they need to get up and move as well as all of the other information it provides not losing more weight than those who don't have that? Using the information that we have already gone over in this book it might be easy to come up with an answer to that.

We know that people are pretty bad at self-reporting their calorie intake, and most of these studies rely on that to follow the participant's diets. What else have we learned about fitness trackers and their calorie counts? They are not all that accurate! So if the participants were relying on their fitness trackers to keep track of their calories in vs calories out then they might have been off by 27% or more! Could there be other factors at play here as well? There is always the possibility that participants were rewarding themselves with food for reaching certain calorie counts or step counts on their trackers. If the participant thought that their workout burnt 400 calories when in reality it was significantly less than that then over eating would be an easy thing to accomplish even if they thought they were still within their calorie deficit for the day. On the other side for the participants who did not have the fitness trackers they would have been mostly in the dark when it came to the issues that I stated above. Not having the "precise" data available to them like their fitness tracker counterparts could have resulted in them being more cautious about their calories in vs calories out estimations.

It seems like there is the possibility that too much information might be a bad thing, when that information is not entirely accurate. I still feel that if used correctly a fitness or activity tracker can be a great benefit to those who are looking to get into better shape or lose weight. However you should be weary of the data that is gathered, such as the calorie counter. As it is now you might be safest to just rely on the old fashion way of counting the calories and nutrients you find on the back of your food labels. If you are still interested in using the apps and gadgets to help you track calories remember to always low ball the estimation on the calories burnt and high ball the calories consumed. This is anecdotal but I have found on several occasions that when people use apps to record their food intake they are usually off on their portion sizes. Meaning that they were eating more calories than they were reporting. This is usually user error in not adjusting the portion size in the app to reflect the portion size consumed. If you want to lose weight and get in shape you need to be precise and accurate about your diet and exercise. Don't go by how many calories your activity tracker says you burnt and always double check the calories in number if using an app. Doing so will ensure that you are not being held back by false data.

103

Bro-Spits

Now that we have spent several days learning about going to the gym, vocabulary, and technologies that might aid you along the way; it is time to learn about several routines, and various exercises you might be interested it. The majority of the remainder of this month will be dedicated to topics like the one that we are covering today. Like the other topics covered during this month, it might not be applicable to you at this moment, but developing an understanding about the different routines will help you in the future. We are going to start out with one that you have probably heard about in the past (usually in a joking way), the Bro-Split.

In recent years the Bro-Split has become somewhat of a joke in media and around the gym. Is it really a joke though? Does it serve a purpose? We should start by defining what a bro-split actually is. Unlike other routines that we will be talking about the term bro-split is more of a blanket term used to describe a basic kind of workout and not a specific routine. How it usually breaks down is a person will perform a resistance weight lifting workout 3-5 days a week and focus on 1-2 muscle groups per workout. So it might look something like this. Monday: Chest and Back. Wednesday: Shoulders and legs. Friday: Arms and Abs. As you can see the majority of the major muscle groups are being exercised once per week. That doesn't sound all that bad does it? No real reason for it to become the butt of jokes in the exercise community. The question is though, does it work?

In short, yes. People who perform a standard bro-split will see results in the gym. It is a very popular weight lifting routine because it allows you to get in all of the major muscle groups in a short amount of time. For those who are new to weight training it is a great way to train the whole body without over doing it. There are some short comings when it comes to the bro-split, and depending on your goals it might not be the routine for you. If your goal is to pack on the muscle and strength then this workout will not be for you. It is not that you will not see muscle development from it; it is that you will be limiting yourself by only hitting each muscle group once per week. Our muscles are able to recover from an exercise in about 3 days, so you would be able to exercise each major muscle group two times in a week. When you only exercise a muscle once per week then you are letting it sit on standby for a week when you could be doubling your workout potential.

If you are new to weight training then the bro-split might be a good start for you. Keep in mind though that as you advance you might need to make adjustments and try a different routine in order to meet your goals. Take your time to thoroughly review your goals and see if the bro-split can help you to reach them. If your goal is to just maintain an overall healthy fitness level and you do not want to pack on the muscle then the bro-split might be a good fit!

Yoga

Yoga is something that people seem to either love or hate. Some people might not like it or do not want to try it because they feel that they are not flexible enough to even begin. Or maybe they are put off by the "spiritual" aspect that can sometime accompany yoga practices. We are not going to cover anything pertaining to the spiritual aspect of yoga, only the health and physical benefits; of which there are a lot! Yoga is often portrayed with skinny people in tight spandex athletic gear standing in rows performing various poses and they are all super flexible. For some people that might be exactly what it is like for them, but for most people it is not even close. Your local gyms might offer yoga classes similar to what I described, and you might enjoy going to a class and giving it a try. However a class is not needed! You can perform yoga routines in the comfort of your own home, typically taking up very little space and little to no equipment needed.

So what is yoga? It is an ancient practice of meditation and exercise that has been increasing in popularity around the world for decades. There are many different types of yoga, some focus more on meditation while others focus on flexibility or strength. It is likely that whatever your goals are or what you enjoy, there will be a yoga style to match it. We are going to focus on the style of yoga known as Hatha. This style tends to be the most popular in the United States because it is a combination of many styles with a focus on the physical poses and controlled breathing. The goal of yoga is for you to challenge yourself but to not become overwhelmed by activity. Next we are going to review some of the health benefits and not specific poses.

Yoga can help to develop a focus on your body and its movements, building your mind muscle connection. We have already learned how important the mind muscle connection is to our physical fitness, and yoga could help you to develop it further. The research has shown that people who perform yoga at least once a week for 30 minutes gained less weight during their middle adulthood years and those who began the study as obese lost weight during the study. Researchers attributed the results to both the physical activity of yoga as well as the mindfulness of your health promoted by yoga routines. Studies have also found that those who practice yoga regularly have more muscle strength, endurance, and flexibility than those who live a sedentary life. Furthermore there are heart health benefits as well; yoga has been found to help lower blood pressure levels in people with hypertension.

So it all sounds great doesn't it? Perform a couple of yoga routines a few times a week and you could reduce your high blood pressure and control your weight. This should not come as a surprise to you. We have spent over 100 days learning about the benefits of just being more active, whether that is through exercise or non-exercise movements. Remember back to the section on flexibility, we spoke briefly about the benefits of stretching when it comes to aches and pains. For me personally I have found that spending 10 to 20 minutes a day performing different yoga poses and stretches can greatly reduce back pain I get from sitting at a desk all day as well as the pain I have from old sports injuries.

If you are reading this section and starting to think that yoga might be something that you could try there are a few things to consider. First you need to know that you do not have to be super flexible to begin yoga. Much like everything else in the fitness area you need to start somewhere and that starting point is usually at the bottom. Research some routines for beginners and give them a try. Focus on controlling your breathing and developing your mind muscle connection. When you are performing stretches you should only go to a point where you can feel tightness or mild discomfort in the muscles and joints. It should never hurt! If you are pushing yourself to the point that it hurts then you are going too far and risking injury. At the start that point might not be very far at all, but if you stick with it then you will become more and more flexible overtime. Just like the adaptations your muscles make to become stronger during resistance training, your muscles and tendons will adapt to become more flexible. It just takes time. If you are interested in trying yoga, do some research and find what type is the best match for you. There are millions of resources out there for different routines and stretches. You can attend classes, purchase workout videos, or find free content on the internet using sites like YouTube. No matter which style you decide to try just research it thoroughly first and be sure to take it slow! If you have any concerns please contact your Doctor before beginning a new yoga workout!

105

Aquatic Exercise

Aquatic exercise is a very broad term that covers any physical activity you perform in the water. This can mean swimming laps, aqua jogging, and water aerobics. The list goes on and on. Is aquatic exercise a good alternative to other forms of exercise? Are you able to get in a good workout to improve your physical fitness or help control your weight? What are some of the benefits of exercising in a pool? We are going to answer these questions in this section and depending on your current fitness level you might find a whole new group of exercises to try!

Aquatic exercises can be a good alternative to other exercises such as walking or running. When you are in the water your body becomes buoyant which means that exercising in a pool is non-weight bearing. So for those who have joint problems or pain, exercising in the water will take the pressure off of your joints. This is especially helpful for those who are carrying around a significant amount of extra body weight. Aquatics can provide you with a means to exercise without the joint pain that can come with standard exercising. Additionally when you are in a pool the water will provide resistance to your body as you perform movements. This resistance can help to build both your muscle strength and endurance!

You have many options when it comes to exercising in a pool. Just recreational swimming will burn as many calories as a brisk walk. You can increase your workout to include things like swimming laps, which will provide you with a full body resistance workout as well as a cardiovascular workout! If swimming laps really isn't your style then maybe aqua aerobics will be more to your liking. Aerobics classes can be a great way for you to get a low impact (easy on your joints) full body workout. These workouts are typically led in a class setting and can include standard movements or more upbeat routines set to music.

No matter your current fitness level aquatic exercises could provide you with a workout that will target your whole body and help you to meet several of the fitness components! If you are interested in trying aquatic activities you will need to do a little research and see what might be available to you. Most fitness centers that have a pool offer daily times in their pool that are dedicated to specific activities like free swimming, lap swimming, aqua aerobic classes and so on. You might be able to find a class that suits your needs or if you have a personal pool you can research routines that you can perform at home. It is important to note that there can be some down falls when it comes to aquatic exercises. One of the main issues people have is cost and time. Purchasing and maintaining a personal pool can be very expensive. The cost of joining a fitness center to use their pool can also be expensive for many people. Check around for the best deals when researching your options. The last downside that we are going to talk about is a physical one. Yes swimming provides great muscle and heart exercises but it removes the weight from your bones. We have learned in a prior section that resistance training can help to strengthen your bones, so exercising in a pool will not aid you in increasing your bone density. If bone density is an issue for you please consult your doctor about finding an appropriate activity.

106

Pilates

Pilates is an exercise routine and program that seems like it has been around forever. For most people my age Pilates is something that their parents or their grandparents did, but it is still a popular form of exercise and its focus on the mind muscle connection is causing it to gain in popularity again. Everyone has probably heard about Pilates at some point or another but you might not know what it actually is. In this section we will briefly go over what it is as well as the 7 principles of Pilates.

First up, Pilates was created by Joseph Pilates as an exercise routine that was intended to help war veterans. However after a little while it became popular with the standard exercise crowd as a means to become more fit. The focus of the program is placed on your core muscles and controlling your breathing. Your movements are to be precise and deliberate, so concentration is very important when performing Pilates. It was this focus on concentration and precise movements that earned it the nick name "the thinking person's workout". Pilate routines are typically body weight exercises, meaning that they do not require any extra equipment or resistance. They focus on strengthening your core muscle and improving your balance. They include a variety of sit-up and crunch styled exercises as well as balance, stretches and push-ups. One of the major benefits of Pilates is that you can perform it with a group in a class setting or in your own home without any cost.

Pilates has a focus on 7 basic principles intended to improve your health, fitness, and control over your body. The 7 principles are mind over matter, focusing on every movement your body makes. Breathing, controlling each breath. Centering, focusing on your core muscles then going outward to the rest of the body. Concentration, focusing on what you are doing. Control, developing complete control over your body. Precision, focus on quality of each action performed. Efficiency of movement; flowing from one exercise to the next without pause.

For many of you I am sure it came as a surprise to learn what Pilates actually is. It is a full body program with focus on your core muscles and body control, both things that I have tried to stress their importance in this book. Participating in a Pilates exercise program can have numerous benefits including achieving all of the fitness components. The exercises can be performed in your own home without any need to purchase equipment. Routines can be adjusted to meet your needs and there are numerous free resources and programs available to you if you wish to research them. One of the best advantages to a Pilate's routine is time! I have pressed you in a past section about time management and finding ways to use your time more wisely to prioritize your activity and health. Pilate's routines can be performed in a short amount of time usually ranging from 15 minutes to a half an hour. Do a little research and give a Pilate's routine a shot, you will be surprised at just how good of a workout you can get!

107

Running

We have all seen those people out there all day running for exercise. Many of us have tried to jump start our weight loss or fitness journeys with running, but is it really worth the effort. I hear it all the time from people who are looking to get in shape that they are going to start running; in fact many people find it very enjoyable. It is a low cost physical activity where the only thing you need is yourself and a safe place to run. But what does the research say?

Well the research is pretty clear, running or jogging is an amazing activity to improve your fitness level and reduce your risk of disease and chronic illness. Research has shown that in people who run there was a 45% reduction in risk of death from heart attack or stroke. There was also a 30% reduction in risk of getting pretty much anything else health related. That is a huge reduction in risk! The best part is that these benefits can be seen in people who only run for 5 to 10 minutes a day! Even better is that your pace does not have to be overly fast either, running at only 6 miles an hour can improve your health. That works out to be a pace of 1 mile in ten minutes. So taking 10 minutes out of your day to go for a slow jog could have amazing impacts on your health!

Still not convinced? Further research into runners has shown that they can add up to 3 years to their life. The researchers concluded that running for an hour added about 7 hours to life benefit. However these results did top out at a certain point, so running won't allow you to live forever. The peak benefits top out at around 4.5 hours of running a week. If you break that down to a 7 day week it is just over 35 minutes of running a day, if you want to reach the peak benefits of running. If what you have read has convinced you that maybe some light jogging each day is something that you could get into, remember to take it easy at first. Use your RPE scale to judge your exertion level and build up over a period of a few weeks. This will allow you to get a feel for what your current abilities are and what pace you should try to run at to achieve your RPE goal.

You will need to take some precautions, check your running area for any hazards that could be dangerous. This includes areas where gravel and debris collects on the road or sidewalks. Look for possible tripping hazards or holes you could step in. Wear bright colors if running near a road or on a trail so motorists and others can see you. Finally be sure that you are wearing proper shoes. Improper or worn out shoes can lead to foot pain and eventually foot or joint problems!

Biking

In our last several sections we have gone over several different strength training and cardio fitness routines and programs. You might have found some of them to be intriguing and want to give them a shot, while others might not have found something that fits their likes, ability, or physical limitations. This is where biking comes in! Remember that saying; "it's like riding a bike" well maybe remembering just how to ride a bike is exactly what you need to get yourself in better health!

In the last section we learned all about the great benefits of running. By running at a slow pace for a few minutes a day you could actually add years to your life! But what if you are not able to run yet? Maybe you have issues with your joints, maybe you are still carrying a little too much body fat and running even for short periods of time can become very painful. Riding a bike can give you a similar workout as running with less impact on your joints. You can purchase your own bike and ride around outside and on bike trails, you can purchase a stationary bike and peddle away while watching your favorite show, or you can even use the bikes at the gym. It is important to know that biking can be called other names as well, such as cycling and in gyms it might be referred to as a spinning class. Let's go over some of the benefits to choosing a bike as your form of physical activity.

First we have already briefly mentioned one of the benefits; it can be easier on your joints than running. When we run our feet make impact with the ground and that force travels up from our feet through our knees and back. When you ride a bike you are in a seated position which takes the weight off of your legs. The pedals also reduce the "impact" and provide less stress on your knee joints. You are still able to get a great cardiovascular workout similar running when you exercise on a bike too! Improving your heart health and your circulatory system! You will also find that you are able to increase your muscle strength and endurance in both your leg muscles and your core muscles. Your quads (front of the legs) and glutes (butt) drive the pedals down while your posterior chain muscles (back of the legs) pull the pedals back up. Your core has to work very hard as well in order to keep you balanced on top of the bike! This balance can be beneficial in your everyday life as well. One of the final benefits that come with biking is the ability to strengthen bones. We have learned that resistance training helps to build and strengthen bones, and that other low impact activities like swimming do not provide bone strengthening benefits. Pedaling a bike is a resistance exercise that is also low impact due to your position on the bike and the removal of your body weight on your legs. However the resistance from the pedals impacts your leg bones and promotes growth.

If you are still searching for a physical activity to accompany with your new healthier diet but you experience joint pain then maybe biking is perfect for you! You will be able to build muscle and burn calories without as much pressure on your joints. If you do begin biking be sure to follow the same safety precautions that we reviewed in the running section. Conduct your own research when selecting a bike as well. Match your bike with your needs and where you want to ride. There are bikes specially designed for any terrain or use.

109

Strong Lifts 5x5

We are going to begin going over some specific weight training programs over the next several days. To start we will be going over Strong Lifts 5x5. To be completely up front and honest about this section, I will admit that I do have a bias when it comes to this program. I have used it when I am returning to lifting after some time off or when I am coming back from injury. I have also recommended it to others and have seen people have great success with it. Keep in mind that not all bias is inherently bad but know that as you read through this section I do specifically like this program.

The way this program works is very simple. You have a workout "A" and a workout "B" That you perform in rotation 3 days a week. Each workout A and B has 3 exercises in it that you perform 5 sets of 5 repetitions. Sounds easy enough doesn't it? Workout A consists of squats, bench press, and barbell rows. Workout B has you doing squats, overhead press, and dead lifts. All of the exercises are completed for 5 sets of 5 repetitions with the exception of dead lift which is performed for 1 set of 5 repetitions. You rotate the workouts each week, so let's say you work out on Monday, Wednesday, and Friday. For one week you will do Workout A on Monday and Friday while doing workout B on Wednesday. The following Week you will do Workout B on Monday and Friday while doing Workout A on Wednesday.

Where this program is really helpful to those who are just starting out or getting back into lifting weights is how low you start with the weights and the gradual application of progressive overload. If you are new to the weight lifting then the program will recommend that you begin using as low of weights as possible. This is usually just the empty bar which is 45 pounds at your standard gym. The benefit of starting so low is that you do not expose yourself to as much risk of injury, you can reduce the effects of DOMS and it gives you time to practice the correct form for each exercise. When you are able to complete 5 sets of 5 repetitions for an exercise then the next time around you will add 5 pounds of weight to the bar, for dead lifts you will add 10 pounds to the bar. Over a short period of time the weight that you are lifting will increase very rapidly and with it so will the difficulty of the workout. When you start the program the exercises will feel very easy but within a month you could be lifting 60 more pounds with your squat and dead lift as well as performing the other lifts with 30 more pounds of weight. As you increase the weight your muscles will become stronger and you will burn more calories. Eventually you will get to a point where the weight is too heavy to complete your 5 sets of 5 reps and when that finally occurs, you do not add any more weight. The next time you attempt the exercise you will try that weight again and if failure continues to happen then the weight will be decreased by 5 pounds and you will try to work up again. Failures happen with this program so do not get discouraged when they do. Keep working hard and you will see results!

The creator of the program has also released a free app that you can use to track your progress. The app is well designed and will automatically increase or keep the weight the same for your next workout depending on how you did in the prior one. What are some of the short comings of the program? To start you are not performing a wide range of exercises. Now this is both a positive and a negative. The exercises being performed are targeting the large muscle groups of the body, which means that you are going to activate a lot of muscle while completing it, which in turn burns calories. However only doing the same handful of exercises can become boring. On the other hand the 3 exercises are an efficient use of muscle and time. You can get a great workout in without spending a large amount of time at the gym. The lifts used in the program require you to use the free weights not the machines. This can be intimidating for some people, but if you take it slow and focus on completing the exercises with proper form your fear of the free weights will be gone in no time.

You will not be able to remain on the program for life; eventually you will hit a peak. I have seen some people remain on the program for months or even up to a year before moving on to another program. I highly recommend it to anyone who is just starting out, but like always consult your doctor before beginning any program. Do your research and see if it is something that you might want to give a try. Remember this program can give great results for both men and women!

110

HIIT

Today is going to be a nice short section for you. We are going to cover HIIT, which stands for High Intensity Interval Training. It is likely that you have heard of this style of workout at some point recently. It was among the most popular fitness trends of 2017. But what is it and what are the benefits performing a HIIT program?

The name says it all, high intensity interval training. You perform an exercise at a very high intensity, usually around 90-95 percent of your maximum ability. Something like a 9 or 10 on your RPE scale. These exercises can range from sprinting to push-ups and weight lifts, as well as burpees and jumping jacks to name just a small amount. You perform the exercise for a short period of time usually around a minute then you rest for a minute or less then you perform another exercise at a high level of intensity. The goal is to get you heart rate up to almost your max heart rate then briefly rest and repeat.

Some research has claimed that HITT training is able to temporarily boost your metabolism. They believe this is done because HITT training increases the oxygen need of our bodies and we will have an oxygen shortage following the workout. The idea here is that our bodies will continue to burn the oxygen after the workout is completed and thus resulting in more calories being burnt. The idea is known as EPOC, excess post-exercise oxygen consumption. Other research has shown that those who participate in HITT workouts lasting around 20 minutes were more motivated and enjoyed the program more than those who completed standard cardio workouts like biking for 20 minutes or more. The participants also showed better physical results than their biking counter parts.

I do not recommend those who are just starting out with physical activity participate in HITT programs right away.

Give yourself some time to become more familiar with exercise and to build your mind muscle connection. This will ensure that you are able to complete various exercises with proper form; reducing your risk of injury. If you think that you would like to try a HIIT workout, like the other ones, do your research and find a plan that fits your needs and goals. I highly recommend that you consult your doctor prior to attempting a HIIT workout to check that your heart is healthy enough for such intense activity.

111

PPL

The next exercise program that we are going to go over is the PPL, or the push, pull, legs program. It is one of the more popular lifting programs that you will find in the gym today. It can be great for both beginners and those who are more advanced; it is often common for those who were doing strong lifts 5x5 to switch to a PPL program as their next phase in lifting. We will go over what makes the program popular and if it is as effective as people like to believe it is.

To start with the basics a PPL program breaks your muscles down into 3 groups. A group of muscles that perform pushing motion; pushing a weight out and away from the body. Muscles that perform a pulling motion; pulling the weight towards the body. Then the last group is the legs group, which is any exercise that focuses specifically on the muscles of the legs. Each muscle group is the central focus of a workout, so for one workout you will only perform exercises that work the pushing muscles and for another workout you only perform exercises for the pulling muscles and so on. This style of exercise is very efficient because there can be a lot of overlap between muscles in each group, while not activating the muscle in the other groups. For example if you are performing the bench press then you are mostly using your chest muscles to move the weight, however your triceps are also being used to help extend the arms at the elbow. This means that you are working both your chest and your triceps in one exercise because they are both pushing muscles. Pulling exercises such as the machine row will work our back muscles primarily but your biceps will also assist in flexing your elbows. This means that you will perform exercises that target each muscle in each group but all of the muscles in that group will be worked out to some extent for each exercise.

This efficiency in exercise selection allows you to get more out of your workout than a standard program like the bro-split. More efficient movements mean that you are going to be building more muscle and burning more calories with each workout. It is pretty easy to see that a PPL program can be broken down into 3 workouts a week. Perform the exercises for each of the 3 muscle groups 1 day a week with a rest day in between each workout day. However this program can also be taken a step farther and be completed 6 days a week with the 7th day being for rest. Essentially it can become a PPLPPL program, and provide you with more opportunity to build muscle and burn calories per week. Why does this work so well for this program? It is simple, as you have learned each exercise day works out a specific group of muscles and those muscles are not activated on the other days. This means that they are able to get plenty of rest before their workout comes up again. For example if you were to do a PPLPPL program starting on Monday and going through Saturday then you would do your push group on Monday and then again 3 days later on Thursday, giving your muscles enough time to recover.

If your goal is to "get the most bang for your buck" then a PPLPPL workout might be the best option for you. Performing this program 6 days a week will allow you to hit each of the muscle groups twice a week. Think about it this way if you performed a standard 3 day PPL program every week for a year then at the end of the year you will have hit each muscle group 52 times individually. Now if you were to perform a PPLPPL program every week for a year then you will have hit each muscle group individually 104 times. That doubles the amount of work and calories burnt in the same time frame. However that does not necessarily mean that you will double your results but you should still get more from it. That being said I do not recommend that you start out with a PPLPPL program, the amount of work load could be too much for a beginner and you will risk extreme DOMS and potential injury. Begin slowly and build into it if you wish to complete a PPLPPL.

Keep in mind though that a standard PPL plan is great for both beginners and those who are more advanced. Take some time to research some of the exercises in a PPL plan and see if it is something that you might find enjoyable. Remember that if you pick a plan you are not stuck with it for years. If you have started another plan and decided that you do not like it or it is too much for your current fitness level, don't be afraid to try a different plan. You need to find something that suits your goals, current fitness levels, time, and life style.

Full Body Split

We have now covered several different workout programs; some require a lot of time and equipment while others don't. What if you want to get in the gym and lift weights but you really don't have that much time to spare. I know I have harped on the idea that you have more time than you think but the truth is that sometimes you just do not have much time to squeeze in a gym workout. Sure you can perform a workout like Pilates at home but maybe you are really trying to make lifting at the gym your go to exercise and use those other options in between. If this describes you then maybe a 2 day full body split is what you need.

What this breaks down to is a simple workout that that you do twice a week on nonconsecutive days, so like a Tuesday and Thursday. Usually these workouts are divided up in one of two ways. One method is that you do a workout that hits all of the major muscle groups for both the upper and lower body in each of the two workouts. The other method is to divide the workouts into two groups an upper body routine completed on the first day and a lower body routine completed on the 2nd day. So for day one you will work out the major muscle groups of the upper body like your chest, shoulders and back. Then for the second workout you will perform lifts for the muscles of the legs such as the quads, hamstrings and glutes. It is a very simple workout routine that you can customize to meet your needs and time. It is also a great way to ensure that you are not leaving out any muscle groups and developing a muscle imbalance or looking like those guys that have 20 inch biceps and 8 inch quads because they always skip leg day.

If you are someone struggling with time or don't want to commit that much time at the gym give a 2 day split a try. It will not take much of your time per week, usually only an hour to an hour and a half total, and you can strengthen all of the major muscle groups of your body. You will also find a boost in your calories burnt aiding you in your weight loss or weight management.

113

Protein Shakes and Weight Loss

Ok so you have decided to take my advice and start working out to help boost your weight loss and overall health. Is it time for you to start drinking protein shakes to make sure you are getting all of the nutrients your muscles need to grow and develop? If you go into any gym you are going to see people drinking their various protein shakes and pre-workouts in an attempt to get the edge they need to build the most muscle and burn fat. But is that something that is actually going to help you on your weight loss journey? Do you need to consume all of that stuff to make sure that your muscles are getting what they need to grow?

No. Well that was simple enough wasn't it? Protein shakes can be very helpful for people to aid in muscle development but they are far from needed. If a person is trying to gain muscle through weight training and increasing their protein intake then they can do so by upping the amount of protein that they consume in their regular everyday diet. Yes protein shakes can help you to get a quick shot of protein to aid in muscle growth but it is far from required. Now let's look at it from the side of weight loss.

Given what we already know about weight loss and what you have likely experienced so far; what do you think adding a protein shake in with your workout is going to do? The answer is very simple. You will increase your calorie intake! I have been practically screaming at you that if you increase your calorie intake your weight loss will either reverse or slow down. So if your goal is to lose weight then why would you want to increase your calorie intake? The short answer is you wouldn't, but you might be concerned that you're not going to get the nutrients your muscles need now that you're working out. Well if that is your concern then you do have a few options. First you can factor a protein shake into your daily calorie intake and cut other food out to make up for the increase in calories. This can be known as meal replacement, where you replace one of your meals with a protein or other shake. The problem with this is that you might become hungry as the shake is digested quicker than a standard meal. Which in turn could lead you to wanting to eat more and inadvertently increase your calorie intake.

Your other option is to increase your daily percent value of protein in your normal diet. This is pretty easy to figure out but you will need to do a little math. First when you want to build muscle it is recommended that you consume between 1 and 1.5 grams of protein for every pound of body weight that you have. For example a 200 pound person should consume between 200 and 300 grams of protein a day when trying to build muscle. Keep in mind that there are 4 calories per gram of protein so you still need to monitor your calorie intake with your increase in protein consumption. The long short of it is that you do not need to fall for the idea that you cannot build muscle without drinking a protein shake. If you are concerned about your protein intake with exercise then consult your doctor and make adjustments to your daily diet to increase your protein intake.

114

Heavy Bag Training

Maybe lifting weights and running isn't your kind of workout. Maybe you like to perform something a little more intense or interactive. Heavy bag boxing training might be a good fit for you. Many people turn to heavy bag training for several reasons, they are relatively inexpensive to purchase and put up in your own home. You can work out on your own time in your own home. You develop cardiovascular endurance and muscle strength as well as muscle endurance. There are all sorts of benefits to trying a heavy bag workout.

If you have every tried a punching bag workout then you will know that it is a very demanding activity. Your heart will be pounding; your arms are going to be exhausted. Your core muscles are going to be tired and your back muscles might become a little sore. You will find that heavy bag training can be a HIIT activity where you perform the exercise of hitting the bag at a high intensity level for a minute or 2 at a time followed by a brief rest period. This type of exercise will increase your heart rate to your target heart rate zone or higher and maintain it there for an extend period of time, resulting in an increase in your cardiovascular endurance. The action of extending your arms out to strike the bag and returning them to your body will use both your pushing and pulling muscles resulting in a muscle strengthening exercise. It is a high impact activity meaning that your body will increase your bone strength and density as you strike the bag and move around the bag. For many people it can also be a major stress reliever and as your core muscles strengthen your balance will improve.

What do you need to consider if you want to try this type of exercise? First and foremost are the safety concerns. They do not call them heavy bags for no reason, they are very heavy and risk of injury to your hands and wrists is a very real possibility. It is not uncommon for someone who does not have the proper equipment or knowledge of the activity to cause injury to themselves. Be sure that if you are going to try this type of exercise that you thoroughly research it and follow the safety guidelines. If you are able to take a couple of classes on how to properly train on a heavy bag I would highly recommend it. Using the proper weight of bag, the correct gloves, and proper wrist protection could keep you from becoming injured during your workouts. It is not just throwing punches as hard and fast as you can either! Take the time to learn the skills needed to do the activity correctly and safely. Like the other programs do your research and take the proper precautions. As always consult with your doctor to make sure that your heart is healthy enough to perform the activity!

115

Couch to 5k

One of the most popular programs I see out there is the Couch to 5k program. The name pretty much gives you all the details about what the programs intended purpose is. It is meant to take a person who either has never been a runner or who might not be in good cardiovascular shape and build them up to be able to run a full 5k. So it takes someone who "sits on a couch" and provides training to get them to be able to run 5 k, which is 3.1 miles. For many people being able to run a 5k is an achievable goal, but not everyone knows how to go about achieving it. So does couch to 5k work? How long does it take? What kind of workout does it give you?

For most people who want to go from not running to being able to run a 5k their training plans consist of going for a run as far as they can then repeat until they get to 5k's. Sure that strategy can work but many people will find it hard to stick to that training plan. The couch to 5k program takes a different approach, one which uses a method we have covered already. The typical plan with the program is to run using the principles of interval training. We have heard that term before haven't we? The couch to 5k plan follows the guideline of HIIT, high intensity interval training. You will run at a variety of speeds followed by periods of walking. Over time the time spent at the faster running pace increases and the time spent at slower paces decreases. The programs usually run 9-12 weeks in length and by the end you should be able to run a full 5k without having to stop or walk.

Now we know from our section on HIIT that interval training is a great way to get your heart rate up for extended periods of time. With the couch to 5k program you are doing just that but it is all through running. The idea is that you will get your heart rate into your target heart rate zone, which will increase your cardio endurance, and your body will adapt to different running paces. So does the program work? It can. Many people have found success using the program but like all exercise programs you have to do it right and put in the appropriate amount of effort. It might be difficult at first but if you follow the guidelines you will see success!

To begin the program you can download the app on your smart phone or there are downloadable hard copy plans that you can use. One of the best parts of the program is its simplicity, just download the program and do what it says every day. The program will tell you how long to run at each pace or how long to walk and all you have to do is put in the effort and follow along. If you are someone who might be interested in running distance runs then this program might be a great way to get you to where you want to be! Just remember to follow the safety guidelines and discuss it with your doctor first, you know the drill by now!

116

Zumba

Zumba quickly became one of the most popular exercise classes in the world. Its upbeat music and use of dance moves to get you up and moving helped to make working out feel less like exercise and more like a dance party. Many of you might have already tried this exercise routine or have wanted to try it but never got around to it. It's popularity might have spiked a year or two ago but it is still a popular exercise program that you can do at many fitness centers or you can perform the routines at home while watching it on video. What is Zumba and what kind of workout can you expect?

There are several different types of Zumba, there is the standard dance class, aquatic Zumba in a swimming pool, or Zumba with weights. For this section we are going to be talking about the standard Zumba class. The concept is that you will follow a choreographed dance that emphasis's moving with the music and just having a fun time. If you are rhythmically challenged like me, you don't have to worry. The moves are easy to follow along with and dancing skills are not required! The program uses interval training where sections of the dance are requiring a higher intensity followed by a lower intensity. As we know this is a great way to elevate your heart rate and keep it up without tiring you out to quickly. You are able to "catch your breath" during the lower intensity sections and give it your all during the more strenuous high intensity sections.

The workout can be considered high impact as you are dancing around and putting pressure on your joints through stepping, bouncing, and jumping. The classes are great for both beginners and those who are more physically fit, no experience is needed. On top of that, outside of a good pair of shoes no equipment is needed. The dances usually focus on developing your cardiorespiratory endurance and burning calories through movement. The muscles targeted are your core and back muscles as well as your legs and glutes. If you are interested in giving the program a try you can start by finding some free routines on the internet or check out a class at your local fitness center. If you are someone who enjoys dancing or would like to have a high energy workout to stay motivated then Zumba could be just the workout for you!

117

P90X

Keeping with our trend of reviewing specific programs we are going to cover one that is a little more difficult, P90X. This program has released at least 3 different versions but we are going to discuss the original program for this section. The program claims that it is for anyone of any fitness level, however this program is hard. Although it can be modified and modifications are shown on the videos, I would not recommend that you jump straight into this program as your very first exercise choice. Don't get me wrong it is a great program that will get you to where you want to be in all 5 of the fitness components, but you might want to work on some basic strength and cardio building exercises before you begin this one.

With the warning and recommendations out of the way let's get into what P90X is. It is a high intensity workout that focuses on strength training, cardio, and flexibility that you can do in the comfort of your own home. The program runs for 90 days and requires a big time commitment from you. You will work out 6 to 7 days a week for an hour or an hour and a half at a time. The program is on 12 different DVDs that it has you complete in a specific order. Some of the workouts focus on strength building while others do cardio routines like plyometric and kickboxing. There are also core routines and flexibility workouts. Now we know what is in the program how does it work? It is pretty simple; you get the DVDs with a workout plan that takes you through 90 days. The workout plan will tell you what workouts to perform on what days, and all you have to do is follow along.

The program also operates on a version of HIIT, where you engage in high intensity activities followed by periods of rest. If you begin this program you will be hitting all of your major muscle groups while also increasing your cardiorespiratory endurance as well as your flexibility. You will need a few things though! Some equipment such as resistance bands some weights and possibly a pull up bar. You can use the resistance bands in place of the pull up bar. The exercises use some weights but they are not required, performing them with just your body weight will still get you results. You will also need a nice clear area to complete the workouts, you will be moving a lot so be sure that the area is clear and free of any hazards you could hurt yourself with.

I do believe that this program is a great one. It is very difficult and will require a time commitment from you. There is a shorter version known as P90X 3 that has 16 workout DVDS that are only 30 minutes in length, so if this type of program peaks your interest there are options available to you. I recommend that if you are planning on trying this workout to perform some basic strength exercises such as daily push-ups and cardio exercises for a few weeks first. This will prepare your body and muscles for the higher intensity workouts in this program. Research the program thoroughly and be sure that it is something that you would like to do, look at each of the versions of the programs and select the one that best matches your needs and goals! If you have been increasing your activity level and performing some exercises over the last 117 days since starting this book then you might be ready to begin this program now, if you would like to.

118

Treadmills

Treadmills have been around for a very long time now and many of you reading this book might already own one. They are a great tool for you to be able to get in a good cardio workout or just get up and get moving inside your own home or in the comfort and safety of a fitness center. One of the major issue is do they actually work? Are they comparable to running outside? And do I need to take the clothes I have had hanging on it for the last 6 months off before I start using it?

The answer to all 3 of those questions is yes, especially that last question; for safety! Treadmills come in all sorts of shapes and sizes now with varying degrees of bells and whistles you can use during a workout. The basic designs have a motor that runs the belt path you walk on at a speed that you select on the control display. Most have the ability to increase the incline to simulate going up a hill and provide you with a harder workout. You just simply set your speed and incline then start walking or running for a period of time. So what are some of the benefits to using a treadmill instead of just going outside and running? Well the easy answer is that you do not have to deal with the elements or safety concerns that accompany running outside. You don't have to worry about the heat, cold, wind or rain. Day light or dark will not matter and you do not have to keep an eye out for potential hazards such as vehicles and tripping risks. A treadmill provides less impact on your knees and other joints compared to running outside as well, and this could be good if you have joint issues. Pacing can be an issue for some people, especially those who are new to running or walking for exercise. It is easy when exercising outside to slow down gradually during your workout without realizing it, on a treadmill you are able to set a pace and leave it there. Many treadmills come pre-programmed with workouts or you can create your own. This means that if you wanted to try HIIT workouts on the treadmill you would be able to. Just adjust the

pace and incline to increase or decrease the intensity. One of
the final major advantages to a treadmill is that you can get a
workout in while also catching up on your favorite shows. Just
turn them on and get moving while you watch!

Some of the disadvantages that you need to keep in
mind if you're planning to go the treadmill route is that you
might not be working out as hard as if you were running
outside. This is because with standard running you have to
propel yourself forward using the muscles of your legs. While on
a treadmill part of that work is done for you by the moving of
the belt under your feet. Wind resistance can also be a factor.
Outside you are running in the air and wind, this provides a
resistance against your body. It might be a large resistance or it
could be very small, either way it is a resistance that is not
present when you are running in place on a treadmill. This boils
down to one important factor, you might not burn as many
calories will running on a treadmill as you would running
outside. However there is a way that you can make adjustments
to counter this! Try increasing the incline on your treadmill so
that you are going slightly up hill. Even a small increase of the
incline will increase the difficulty of the workout and therefore
increase the total calories burnt!

Other issues that you need to be aware of are located
on many treadmills themselves. I mentioned that some
treadmills come with different bells and whistles that you can
use during your workout. One of the most common ones is a
calorie function. This function tells you how many calories you
are burning during your workout. What have we learned about
these types of counters? That's right; they are not very accurate
or reliable. They are typically just estimations and do not take
your height and weight into account, which is needed to
estimate your calories. Even if your treadmill does take your
height and weight into account it is still very likely that it will not
be accurate. Play it safe and do not try to use the calories burnt
number provided by the treadmill to estimate your daily calorie
needs. You might end up not burning as many as you thought;

which will slow down your weight loss if your increase your calorie consumption based on daily calories burnt.

All in all a treadmill can be a great exercise tool to help you get into better shape and lose weight. You can make adjustments to the speed and intensity of your workout to make it harder or easier. Continue to use your RPE scale to estimate how much effort you are putting into your workouts. Also keep in mind that all of your activities do not have to be high up on your RPE scale, sometimes just a nice slow paced walk is all you need. Any activity is better than no activity! If a treadmill is an option for you, you might want to give it a try a couple times a week.

119

Balance/Exercise Balls

We have discussed balance balls in prior sections before and how you can use them to increase your muscle engagement while sitting, but there is a lot more that you can do with them! This will be a short section where we go over some of the other uses of balance balls, also known as exercise balls. You might be surprised to find out that they can be used for more than just bouncing on.

First we have already gone over that sitting on an exercise ball can help you improve your balance as well as burning more calories than just sitting in a standard chair. This happens because you have to make constant adjustments to remain balanced on the ball by activating the muscles in your legs and core. However there are other uses for them that can aid you in standard workouts as well as provide alternatives to other exercises. It is recommended that if you are new to using an exercise ball that you spend a little bit of time just sitting on it and moving around slightly. This will allow you to get a feel for how the ball moves and what sort of adjustments you will need to make in order to remain balanced during an exercise. One of the more common uses for the exercise ball is to aid in core exercises. You can lay your back across the ball and plant your feet in a comfortable position. Once you find your balance you can perform crunches and sit-ups on the ball, as well as, a variety of other core strengthening exercises. The benefits of performing these actions on the exercise ball can include reducing the stress your spine as well as allowing you to increase your range of motion during an exercise. By this I mean that when you are doing a standard crunch on the floor you can only go back until your back is flat against the ground. When you are on the exercise ball you can go further by arching your back along the curve of the ball. This will force your core muscles to have to contract for a longer distance, giving them a longer workout.

You can also use the balance balls during other exercise to improve your posture. For example, if you are performing a dumbbell shoulder press; which is when you take a dumbbell and press it straight up over your head, you need to keep your back straight. When doing this exercise standing or sitting on a standard bench then you might slouch or arch your back. This can lead to back pain or injury! Performing the exercise while sitting on a balance ball will help you to keep your spine in line and have good posture, reducing your risk of injury. This is done because you will need to keep your back straight to balance the ball while pressing the weight up.

I could spend dozens of pages going over the various exercises that can be adapted to use the exercise ball with, but that is not the purpose of this book. I encourage you to research some of the options provided by incorporating exercise balls into your workouts. If you decide to add some of the exercises to your routine be sure to do so safely. Follow all safety guidelines and take it slow. If your balance is not all that great you should work on improving it before you try to sit on a balance ball and press a weight up over your head or perform other exercises! Adding a balance requirement to your exercises increases your risk of injury! Be safe, because an injury would set your progress back by weeks or months!

120

4 Months in, 2 to Go

Can you believe that it has been 4 months already? We are at day 120! Have you been seeing some progress? If you have been counting your calories and watching your portion sizes as well as increasing your activity level you will have seen some results by now. You might not be at your goal weight yet, but you are on your way! If you have already reached your goal I recommend that you continue reading until the end, there are things that you will learn that will help you to maintain at your goal weight for life!

Now that we are entering into a new month and completed two thirds of this book you should take the time to reassess your TDEE and make any dietary and activity adjustments to keep yourself on track. If you have already reached your goal weight then you should check your TDEE to see how many calories your body uses in a day. You can increase your calorie intake so that you are no longer at a deficit and enter your maintenance phase where you consume at or around the same amount of calories as you burn during the day. If you have not met your goal weight yet then you should continue to operate at a calorie deficit and consider increasing your percentage of calories cut. Remember you should be cutting 15-25 percent of your TDEE calories each day.

At this point I hope that you have increased your activity level. This can mean increasing your NEAT levels or increasing your activity through exercise. It is important for you to remember that you cannot outrun a bad diet! This means that even though you might be exercising you will not lose weight without getting control of your diet! Keep making healthy food choices and monitoring your nutritional intake. This will lead you to success and allow you to maintain long term weight loss!

Keep up the great work, the changes that you have made should be starting to become second nature. You have been slowly changing your old habits and replacing them with more healthy habits that will promote weight loss and improve your overall health. Keeping this up for 4 months is a huge accomplishment! Remember that most diets fail after only 5 weeks! We have been at it now for over 17 weeks! That is something to be proud about, take today to reflect on how far you have come, and don't be afraid to pat yourself on the back.

You should also take today to reassess your goals. Since you first started this journey and created these goals it is possible that they have changed. Look at the goals you have set, and make adjustments if they have changed over the course of the last 4 months. If they haven't check to see that you are still on track to achieve them in the time frame that you wanted to! You might need to make adjustments to your behavior in order to reach your goal or you might need to make adjustments to your time frame!

Keep up the great work and keep reading, there is still more that you can learn.

121

Strength Training Means You Have to Lift Heavy Weights

There is an idea out there that if you want to strength train that you have to go to the gym and lift heavy weights. The truth is that this is a myth! Strength training comes in many forms and can be tailored to fit your individual goals. In fact you don't need to lift weights at all to strengthen your muscles. There are methods, strategies, and workouts out there to suit basically any goal and to do so through a variety of methods.

Now being realistic if you want to look like a bodybuilder then you are likely going to have to pick up some heavy weights for a few sets, but if your overall goal is to build up your muscle strength then there are other ways! First we have already discussed this a little in an earlier section, building strength and muscle can be done through lifting lower weights for higher reps. Our bodies are amazing and will adapt to the stresses that we place on them. If you have ever tried weight lifting then you know that the heavier the weight the harder it is to lift, that's some basic science right there. However if you have ever taken a lighter weight and tried to lift it for more reps you will find that it can be equally as difficult. You might be able to achieve the same muscle fatigue lifting a 35 pound weight 8 times as you do by lifting a 25 pound weight 15 times. Some research has shown that when experienced lifters were divided into two groups those who did lower weight and higher reps developed similar amounts of muscle mass as those who performed higher weights and lower reps. In my opinion this works well for beginner's and casual lifters, so for the average person lifting lighter weights for strength, more reps will give you similar results as lifting heavier weights.

There are other options available to you as well, ones that leave the weights in the gym. Bodyweight exercises are growing in popularity and were one of the most searched exercise routines of last year. Body weight exercises can include your basic push-ups or pull-ups, squats and planks, they can also become more advanced and more difficult as you become stronger and increase in fitness. Many people have found great success by performing body weight exercises and routines. The best part about these exercises is that your own body and gravity provide the resistance. So there is no need to purchase other equipment! We have already reviewed a handful of body weight exercises and routines. Push-ups and sit-ups were covered early on while more recently we have discussed yoga and Pilates.

If you are still apprehensive about trying resistance training because you are discouraged by the heavy weights or your inability to lift them, I hope this section helped you to get passed that. Strength training is any activity that strengthens your muscles! You can accomplish this by lifting any weights as long as you are pushing yourself hard enough to force your body to adapt to the stress, or you can achieve this by simply performing exercises that use your bodyweight as the resistance to your muscles. The gym or expensive equipment can help you but ultimately they are not needed. All that is needed is your willingness to push yourself and force your body to adapt and change!

122

Altitude Training Masks

It is no secret that athletes and those looking to get fit like to try and find short cuts. Whether those short cuts promise to increase your results by more than the other guy or by speeding up your weight loss, short cuts are promoted everywhere. We are going to take a moment and look at one such short cut in the cardio training world. Altitude Training Masks.

You might have seen these devices on TV, in advertisements or in use by people. Their intended purpose is to make it harder for you to get oxygen into your body and therefore forcing your body to become more efficient and increase your cardiorespiratory endurance. It is meant to simulate training at a higher altitude. So basically it makes it harder to breathe while you work out. But, does this have any basis in science or is it just more quackery?

Ok, so we know that different altitudes above sea level have different levels of oxygen. The higher up you go the less oxygen you can bring in per breath. The body has a natural response to this, people who live at or train in higher elevation areas increase the number of red blood cells that they have. We know that red blood cells carry oxygen throughout the body to where it is needed. When at a higher elevation where the air is thinner your body will increase its red blood cell count in an attempt to be more efficient with the lower oxygen levels. The long short of it is that the more red blood cells you have the better your cardiorespiratory endurance will be. Athletes will try to force their bodies to increase their red blood cell count by training at higher elevations and then competing at lower elevations. This technique means that they will have more efficient cardiorespiratory systems that can provide more oxygen to their muscles especially at lower levels of elevations. You might have heard issues involving this in various sports; two good examples are Mile High Stadium in football. The home field of the Denver Bronco's is at a high elevation, so when the away team plays there they might be at a disadvantage because their bodies are not prepared to perform with less oxygen. Another example is in the world of cycling. You hear about it often that bike racers might be blood doping. This is the practice of adding more blood to the body usually through an IV. So they are artificially increasing their red blood cell count through external means and improving their performance.

The science supports the idea that reducing your oxygen intake leads to increases in red blood cell count, and the increase in red blood cells leads to better cardio endurance. So the mask sounds like it will help to give people an edge. Well it doesn't. The major problem with the mask is that it just restricts your breathing resulting in not being able to get air into your lungs at your normal rate. This works on two systems of your body, your inhale and exhale. The level of oxygen molecules that are in the air are the same when you wear the mask. So each breath provides the same amount of oxygen, the only difference is that it is harder to get the air into your body. As a result it is also harder to get air out, meaning that you're going to have a build-up of CO_2 in your blood system. CO_2 is a waste product created by our body systems and removed through our respiratory system. Restricting your breathing during exercise will make you feel fatigued or "winded" sooner. Because of this you might think that the mask is working for its intended purpose but this simply is not true.

Now that is not to say that the altitude masks provide benefits in other areas. If your goal is to look like the Batman villain Baine while you work out then you will certainly achieve that! It is possible that because the mask makes it harder to breathe in and out it will strengthen your muscles that control your breathing. It is important to note that strengthening these muscles will not have effects on your athletic performance. In the end I do not see any reason for you to consider trying one of these masks in an attempt to take a short cut. Hard work will get you the results, not buying some special product with inflated claims.

123

Sweating is a Good measure of a Workout

I recently saw a deodorant commercial that featured a bunch of high school guys at sports practice. The coach was putting them through a workout and all of them but one was sweating profusely. The coach told the kids that no one gets a drink until the one kid that wasn't sweating finally broke a sweat. This follows the idea that if you're not sweating during a workout you're not working hard enough. But is this idea true?

You might be surprised by the answer, no it is not true. I guess you probably were not surprised at all. Sweating is something that we all do during the whole day; it is a natural response to heat and other factors like humidity. When your body heats up it will release sweat through its 4 million sweat glands. This doesn't mean that you will release the same amount of sweat as the other guy. Factors such as gender, age, weight, and fitness level can determine how much you sweat. It is true that the harder you work out the more your body will heat up and as a result you are more likely to sweat but there can be other factors such as the outside temperature. You are likely going to sweat more running in 90 degree weather than you will running on a treadmill in a 68 degree gym. Your hydration level can also influence the amount you sweat. If you become dehydrated then your body will reduce the amount of sweat that it releases in an attempt to preserve water.

In the end you should not use your level of sweating to tell how hard you are working out. We have already gone over a method for you to gauge your activity effort. The Rate of Perceived Exertion scale, or RPE. If you have not tried using this scale during your workout I recommend going back to the section we covered it in and review it. The RPE scale allows you to estimate how hard you are working during exercise. The best part of the scale is that the numbers remain the same as your fitness increases. So a pace for an exercise that use to be really hard for you might become easier for you overtime. As you notice the exercise becoming easier you will notice your RPE number dropping, as a result you will know that you need to increase your effort to keep your RPE at optimal level for your goals.

124

Muscles of the Body: Quadriceps

It is time to take a short break from learning about exercise routines and take a look at a very big important muscle group in our bodies, the Quadriceps, Quads for short. The Quads are the muscles that are on the front of our upper legs. They are one of the largest muscle groups in the body, but the Quads are not one single muscle it is actually made up of 4 separate muscles! They are the Vastus Medialis, Vastus Lateralis, Vastus Intermedialis and finally the Rectus Femoris.

The Vastus Medialis is found towards the inside of the leg. It can become very defined towards the knee joint and is sometime referred to as the "tear drop" because of its shape. The Vastus Lateralis is the opposite of the Medialis and can be found towards the outside of the leg. The Vastus Intermedialis is the muscle that sits in between the two muscles just mentioned. It makes up the front part of the thigh. Finally the Rectus Femoris is the narrowest of the Quad muscles and it sits mostly on top of the Intermedialis. All four of the muscles come together into a tendon that attaches at the patella, or knee cap. Your knee cap is a bone that is embedded within the tendon of the Quads. Its function is to keep the tendon from rubbing on the femur as the knee joint bends and strengthens. It also serves to increase the mechanical advantage of the muscles increasing their strength by 20%!

Now that we know what the Quad muscle consists of what is it that it does? Their primary function is to extend the leg at the knee joint. If you are sitting in a chair and kick your leg out by straitening your knee you will have done so by using your Quad muscles. They also serve the function of stabilizing the knee joint and the Rectus Femoris helps to flex the hip. The quads are crucial in activities that include walking, running, jumping, and squatting. Basically any activity that involves your legs extending at the knee joint your quads will be involved. You can specifically exercise your quads through running and lifting exercises such as squats, leg extensions and using the leg press machine. They are a very large muscle group and as such take a lot of calories to maintain them throughout the day. Increasing your quads strength could help to increase the natural amount of calories you burn throughout the day. You might want to consider adding in some Quad training into your workouts!

125

Muscle of the Body: Ham Strings

Yesterday we learned about the major muscle group of the front of the legs. Today we will learn about the major muscle group for the back of the legs, the Hamstrings. The Hamstrings like the Quads are a large collection of muscles located in the upper portion of the back of your legs. There are 6 muscles that are usually associated with the hamstrings. They include the Gluteus Maximus, Adductor Magnus, Semimembranosus, Biceps Femoris, Gracilis, and finally the semitendinosus.

The hamstrings begin or originate at the hip bone and top of the femur then run down the back of your leg behind your knee. They connect at different sections of the lower leg bones named the tibia and fibula; which are below the knee joint. What is it that the hamstrings do? They are used in activities that involve walking, running, and jumping. Specifically they are used to flex the knee joint. This means that they will bring your leg from a straight position to a bent positon at the knee. If you were to bend your leg so that your heel came up towards your butt you would be using your hamstrings. They are the antagonists of the quads, in that they reverse the actions of the quads. In the same sense the quads are the antagonists of the hamstrings.

If you are training your leg muscles it is important that you keep the strength of your quads and hamstrings relatively equal so that they can function together properly. Some good exercises include the squat and dead lift. You should also consider keeping your hamstrings flexible. When we sit our hamstrings are pulled tight and prolonged sitting can cause some hamstring problems and even lead to back pain as the hamstrings become tight and pull of the hips and lower back. Keep in mind that Hamstrings can become injured in activities that require a lot of starting and stopping of running.

Strengthening and stretching of the hamstrings can help to reduce your risk of injury.

In order to maintain good overall health and fitness you should incorporate exercises into your routine that strengthens you hamstrings. This will help you to complete other exercises as well as improve your overall quality of life in day to day tasks. Take some time to research some hamstring exercises and stretches. Increasing your hamstring flexibility could really help to reduce some of the leg and back pain you might currently experience!

126

Balance Boards

Another piece of equipment that has found great popularity in recent years is the humble balance board. We have already learned at length the benefits of balancing with equipment such as the balance ball or balance cushions. What if you are looking for a standing balance exercise? Well then a balance board might be what you are looking for.

First, what is a balance board? The most basic design is simply a firm platform that you stand on with a dome on the underside. This dome makes the board unstable and forces the person standing on it to constantly make adjustments to remain balanced on the board. So basically it serves the same sort of function as the balance balls we have already discussed except you're standing. Are there other benefits that you can receive from using a balance board that you cannot get from a balance ball?

Yes. The reason why there are different or added benefits is pretty simple, you sit on a balance ball and you stand on a balance board. This means that you are using different muscles in an attempt to remain balanced. Standing on a balance board will activate more of your leg muscles including those of your ankles. Using a balance board can greatly improve your coordination. To remain balanced you need multiple muscle groups to work together and function as one. For some people with low coordination this can be difficult, but with proper training you can improve your body's coordination. This can be very beneficial for athletes in sports like football where your goal is to remain on your feet. As we walk and move around throughout the day it is easy to slip or stumble from time to time. When this happens our bodies have to respond very quickly to try to prevent a fall. Using a balance board can help to improve our body's reaction time to events like this.

You can use balance boards in a variety of ways. You can purchase one and use it as part of your daily routine at home or you can use them at the gym. However there has been a rise in popularity in using them at work with standing desks. We have gone over standing at the office before, as well as the effects of sitting for extended periods of time. Due to this it is no wonder that people are turning to simple exercise habits while at work. Working at a standing desk is a great way to keep yourself moving throughout the day and burning extra calories. Adding in the balance board would allow you to work out even more without interfering with your job.

Much like the balance balls it can be very dangerous to use them improperly or outside of a safe area. If you are choosing to add them into your regular routine or as part of your work place activity be sure that you are following all of the safety guidelines and you are able to use it correctly. Like all of the other things take it slow and ease into its use. This will help to reduce your chance of becoming injured.

127

Vegan Diet

Let's take a break from the fitness discussions and turn back to a dietary based subject, the Vegan diet. It is very unlikely that in this day and age you would not have heard at least some details of a vegan diet. It has really gained popularity starting back around 2010, however its origins date back much further. The term Vegan was coined back in 1944 when the Vegan Society was founded in England. This society took on the doctrine that "man should not live by exploiting animals". Which is the center point of today's veganism.

Now that we know a little bit about the history let's review what Vegan actually is. Like all diets there are different versions and Veganism is no exception. For the purpose of this section we will be discussing the basic standard principles of the vegan diet. It really boils down to a stricter form of a vegetarian diet. Recall back to when we covered the vegetarian diet, for the most part people who followed the diet would almost exclusively eat plant based foods. However there were some sects that would still eat dairy and eggs. In a vegan diet there is no animal based products consumed at all; it can also be taken a step further. Most vegans are against any type of product that is created using animals either as a base for the product or in the testing phase.

As we have learned a diet that is heavy in plant based foods has countless benefits for your health and wellbeing. It helps to keep your carbohydrate consumption down as well as fewer foods containing the bad fats. Your blood sugar can remain more stable and your fiber intake is typically pretty high which leads to better digestive health. Some of the down sides are that you might miss out on some of the essential amino acids needed to create protein. Plant based foods contain incomplete amino acids while meat products contain complete amino acids. Because of this people who eat a plant based diet need to ensure that they get a variety of foods to consume all of the amino acids they need throughout the day. Since vegans do not consume any animal products it is important that they monitor their nutritional intake to keep from becoming malnourished.

If a vegan diet sounds like it is something that you would be interested in adopting you should consult with your primary doctor and see what your options might be. It is a lifestyle that has shown to reduce your risk of disease and chronic illness. However you do need to be mindful of the nutritional gaps that you could develop as a result of cutting out major food groups. Like everything else I have mentioned conduct thorough research so that you can make an educated choice that best suits your health and life style.

128

Body Weight Exercises

Let's quickly review a topic that we have covered a few times in other sections but have yet to dedicate a full section to it. That topic is body weight exercises. We have spent time already covering different specific routines such as Pilates or Zumba that use your own body as the resistance to your muscles but are the benefits worth the effort?

When we discuss bodyweight exercises we are talking about any exercise that does not require equipment to provide the resistance. You do not need weights or machines to perform the exercises all you need is your body. Some exercises might need equipment in the form of a pull up bar but even using a pull up bar your own body weight is what is providing the resistance against your muscles not the machine itself. Two of the major benefits to engaging in body weight fitness is that 1 it is free and 2 you can do it anywhere at any time. If you are tight on cash or just don't see the need for spending money on gym memberships or other equipment then bodyweight exercises will provide you with an opportunity to exercise and improve your strength without lightening your wallet. We have already learned that you do not need heavy weights to increase your muscle size or strength. This means that you will be able to improve both just by spending a little time each day working with different bodyweight exercises. If you are like millions of other people around the world you live a very busy life and it can be difficult fitting things into your day. So make body weight exercises just a part of your routine. It should only take you around a minute to complete 30 push-ups. Working in 3 sets of push-ups a day should only take you around 3 total minutes. Do 30 as soon as you get of bed, as you're getting ready for your day do 30 more before you get in the shower, followed by 30 more before you get dressed. See how easy it can be to add in 90 push-ups before you even get to work? Body weight exercises can be a great way to squeeze in a little extra work during the work day and without taking much time. Every hour at work you could stand up and do 10 body weight squats. By the end of a standard day you completed around 80 squats. Add in 3 sets of 30 crunches between your activities at home and just like that you have a 3 bodyweight exercise plan for each day will take up very little of your time.

I provided you with some examples above you can either try to sprinkle some extra activity throughout the day or you can put together a 20 to 30 minute plan to complete a few times a week. Take time to look into all of the different body weight exercises you can try and their variations. Piece together your own routine or look for one that is already created. Adding it in could really boost your calories burnt and get you towards your goal that much quicker!

129

Revisit your Goals

On day 120 I asked you to take some time and look at your goals. You should have been checking to see if those goals were still what you were hoping to achieve or did your goals change? When you are revisiting your goals you should be checking to see if you are going to meet your goal in the time frame that you set for it, or do you need to make an adjustment. For today I want you to really think about what it is that you want to achieve through completing this book.

You might have already achieved your weight loss goal, if you have are you content with where you are or do you think now that you are at your goal weight you could actually go a little further. If you are where you want to be then look into setting goals that could help you for long term maintenance. For example, we know that our weight will fluctuate throughout the day or week. You can set a goal that you will remain within 5 pounds of your goal weight at the end of every month. This way you will check your weight at the end of every month and if you gained then you know that you will need to reduce your calorie count for a little while to remove the weight gain. If you are within your 5 pounds then you know you can continue as you are. Setting goals like this will prevent you from following into that weight loss paradox of losing the weight then returning back to old habits and gaining it all back.

If you have not achieved your weight goal yet do not be discouraged! You have been working towards it now for over 4 months. You should be seeing some results. If you have not been seeing results or not seeing the results that you were expecting then you need to do a few things. First you need to reassess that your goal is realistic. Expecting to lose 50 pounds in a month would not be realistic. However if your goal is realistic and you are not on track for achieving it then you need to reassess your TDEE. Once you know your TDEE cut 15-25 percent off of it and that will give you your total calories you should eat a day. Be sure that you are accurately counting your calories and measuring out your portion sizes. If you are doing all of that correctly you will lose weight.

Take today and really think about what you want and where you would like to be. Remember your journey doesn't end on the last page of this book. You might reach your goal by then or it might still be a ways off. Set your goals to be realistic to what you can achieve in a time frame that you can achieve them! Don't forget to break down your bigger goals into small goals that you can achieve along the way. Don't under sell the importance of small victories to keep you motivated!

130

Challenge Yourself

Far too often people are afraid to step out of their comfort zone and try some new things. This is especially true in the realm of exercise. People find themselves being afraid to even begin an exercise or if they do they will stick with the same one afraid to branch out and try something different. That is the topic of today's section, challenge yourself.

We have been working on making dietary changes and changes to your daily habits that will lead to lifelong success. I have been pushing the concept of adding in physical activity to you daily routines. I have expressed its benefits and provided you with several different examples on various programs and routines that might fit your needs or goals. The problem is that I cannot force you to do any of them! Only you can make the decision to try one of the exercise routines.

Today I want you to take the time to think about an exercise or program that I have suggested or one that you have researched on your own. Consider your goals and what you have achieved so far. Think about what it is that you are good at or comfortable with and apply it to some sort of physical activity. It can be something that you have wanted to do but for whatever the reason you have not mustered up the courage to go through with attempting it. It can just be a random one that you have heard about or one that I have mentioned.

After you have found that exercise or program I want you to just give it a try for a few days. It doesn't have to be today, you can use today to decide on what you want to do. Once you have made your decision just go and do it. Challenge yourself to do the activity for a week or 2 and see how it feels. You just might find that you really enjoy it or that you were avoiding it for no reason! Don't let fear, anxiety, or excuses get in your way. Find something new and give it a try. Take it from a

guy who is terrified of heights but yet became a pole vaulter;
don't let fear stop you from trying something!

131

Obesity: Hypertension

We are on day 131 so I really hope by now I do not need to inform you that obesity can increase your risks for certain illnesses and diseases. That being said there are a few more issues involving obesity's effects on the body that I would like to review. The more you know the better informed decisions you will be able to make that will impact your life long health. In this section we will be covering Hypertension.

Hypertension is just a longer term for high blood pressure. This referrers to the pressure applied to the inner wall of your arteries, and you can be diagnosed with hypertension based on the average of two or more blood pressure screenings. You should know that being Ill or already being on medication that effects your blood pressure during a screening should not be counted in the average when deciding if you have hypertension or not. When you get you blood pressure measured it will be the combination of 2 numbers. One is called the systolic which is the upper number and the diastolic which is the lower number. These numbers will place you into one of 3 categories. Normal Blood Pressure which has a range of the systolic number being at 120 or less and the diastolic number being at 80 or less. Next is the pre-hypertension range which is your systolic number falling between 120-139 and your diastolic number being between 80-89. The final classification is hypertension which is broken down into two sub classification. Stage 1 has a systolic range of 140-159 and diastolic range of 90-99. Stage 2 is anyone who has a systolic at or above 160 and a diastolic at or above 100.

The issues caused by hypertension are too numerous to go over in detail in this book. What you need to know is that overtime high blood pressure can cause your artery walls to become damaged; these damaged areas can become clogged as well as become more ridged resulting in limited blood flow. As the pressure on the artery increases you run a higher risk of aneurysm which is when a weakened artery bulge's out or ruptures cause life threatening injury. Hypertension will increase your risk of coronary heart disease as well. The heart is a muscle and like all muscles it needs blood to function so the heart has to provide itself with blood too. This is done through coronary arteries that run along the heart. When blood cannot flow freely though these arteries, you could experience chest pain or even a heart attack. Hypertension makes it so your heart has to work harder in order to pump blood throughout the body. This can cause your heart to become enlarged specifically the left ventricle. A condition that increases your risk of heart attack, heart failure and sudden cardiac death.

The list just keeps going and includes things like issues with your kidneys, brain, eyes, and even sexual dysfunction. Hypertension is closely linked to obesity. Carrying around excess weight greatly increases your risk of high blood pressure and all of the issues that can accompany it. There is hope though! If you are someone who is/was overweight or obese losing weight has been shown to decrease your blood pressure and could help to reduce your risk of contracting the ailments associated with it. Take the time to get your weight under control and it very well could improve your quality of life in hundreds of ways! If you feel you are at risk of hypertension please seek out medical care immediately.

132

Jumping Rope

When was the last time you jumped rope? It has probably been years, maybe even more years then you care to admit. Jumping rope seems to have two homes, elementary PE class and Rocky Movies. However the jump rope is an amazing piece of workout equipment that could really boost your cardio and weight loss results!

It might sound surprising that jumping rope can be such a great workout considering that most people see it as just a child's toy but in reality it is very versatile and provides a difficult workout. I do not believe that I need to explain what jumping rope is, it is literally all in the name. You jump over a rope you are swinging in rhythm. What you might not know is how many types of jump ropes there are and you can use them for different types of workouts depending on what you prefer. There are your standard beaded ropes that help to keep the rope in a certain shape and more rigid. These ropes are great for beginners as they make it a little easy to keep a rhythm and the rope keeping a wider shape gives you more room for clearance. There are plain rope jump ropes that you can use if you want to go a little faster than the beaded ropes and there are also very thin vinyl jump ropes which offer the fastest rotation. Finally there are some ropes that are more like tubes that are filled with sand. These ropes are slow but provide a lot of resistance to your arms as you swing them.

The benefits from jumping rope, not surprisingly involve a lot of cardiorespiratory endurance development. You will be jumping up regularly while swinging your arms against the weight and air resistance of the rope. On top of the cardio benefits you will also be increasing your muscle strength and endurance. The action of jumping repeatedly will not only increase your muscle strength by pushing yourself up off the ground but during the landing your legs will be slightly bent to absorb the impact. During this absorption on impact your muscles will have to tighten to keep yourself upright, providing more muscle strengthening exercise. The action of rotating the rope with your arms will both improve your shoulder and grip strength but also have the added benefit of increasing your shoulder flexibility.

There are several ways that you can perform a jump rope workout. The most popular method is to do a HIIT workout. Perform timed periods of high intensity work followed by some rest times. If you are new to jumping rope then you can experiment a little with your work/rest times. Start by doing a ratio of 1:1. Do 30 seconds on then 30 seconds off. Slowly work up to a minute on and a minute off then increase your time jumping rope to be greater than your time resting. Slowly you will increase your cardio endurance to the point you can jump for extended periods of time! Do a little research and you will be able to find that you can jump in different ways to increase the difficulty or engage the muscles in a different way. Keep in mind that although it is a jumping exercise, if done properly it is no more high impact on your joints then jogging! Give jumping rope a try, it is a great workout at home or take it with you on the road. If you go on a trip you can easily make room for a jump rope in your luggage!

133

Bring your Whole Family Along for the Journey

For those of you who have families at home, it could be a spouse or kids, you might find greater long term success if you bring them all along for the journey. If your family is dedicated to eating healthier and being more active with you then you will have fewer opportunities for temptations! Research also shows that your choices as a parent can greatly affect your children's health and future.

It is no secret that parents set the standard for their children. Kids like to follow along with what their parents do and imitate what they see. If their parents eat junk food then they will likely eat junk food. If their parents come home from work and plop down of their couch for the rest of the night then they will probably follow suit. Kids pick up our hobbies, likes, dislikes, political ideologies, so it is not hard to imagine that they will also pick up our nutritional and exercise habits as well. Resent research shows that mothers likely have the biggest influence on their child's weight and activity level. Studies have shown that when a mother loses weight the kids lose weight and when mothers eat healthy the kids eat healthy. There was no significant link between the father's health habits and the child. Seems a little unfair doesn't it? Putting all of that pressure and "blame" on one parent! The researchers said that this is likely due to the mothers typically being responsible for activity and meal planning. So it does not specifically effect women greater than men due to biology but more likely due to roles within the family structure. So fathers who plan meals and activities you could be a factor in your child's health as well!

Your family can be a fantastic support structure and if they join you on this journey then you will find that you will have an easier time staying motivated. I am sure that it is no surprise that the research shows when a family or close social circle all follow the same diet or exercise plan all members see greater results then those doing it on their own. This is because of the support structure that you develop. You will have people going through the same issues as you and you will have people to talk to and encourage you along the way. Taking this journey with others is also a great way to hold yourself accountable. Most of the time if your motivation is swaying or you want to give up; the feeling of not wanting to let the others down could be a huge motivator to get you back on track!

Try planning healthy meals that all of the family will enjoy. Slowly replace the junk food in your house with healthy alternatives. This will help in two ways. First your family will become healthier and adopt the healthier habits. Secondly if the junk food is not in the house then that means no one will be able to eat it in front of you! You can plan family activities that involve movement as well. Instead of going to the movies try going to the zoo, there your will be walking and on your feet all day while spending time with your friends and family. Set yourself up for success and your family will follow your lead. You might even be able to set them up for success so that they don't need to read this book in their future! You can be a great example and role model for the generations that follow you. Your children could be healthier resulting in better health for their children and down the line it continues!

134

Crabs in a Bucket

No this section is not on the nutritional benefits of seafood. This is going to be a short section on the phrase "Crabs in a Bucket". The saying refers to the action of crabs when they are trapped in a bucket or pot. A single crab could probably escape the bucket but the other crabs will latch on and undermine their efforts. This prevents any of the crabs from being able to escape or achieve something. So what does this have to do with health and weight loss? More than you might have thought!

Remember how we have learned that most long term weight loss attempts fail? We also have learned how most diets have a run time of about 5 weeks. Now I have covered these issues at length and tried to show why this is. Understanding why so many people gain the weight back within 5 years is a great way for you to know how to prevent it. That being said at this point in time there is are still millions of people out there that will be starting and failing at their diets. They might have achieved some weight loss but are now slowly gaining it back. I don't want to sound too cynical but it is the truth. These failures tie in to the crabs in a bucket metaphor perfectly. When people see others success in areas that they failed there can be a certain "if I can't have it no one can" mentality, even if they don't even realize they are doing it. So undermining your progress and willpower can become their own personal goal. This won't happen to everyone but you will likely find it in a few people you interact with.

You might have already experienced something along these lines. I am sure that you have received your fair share of "congrats" and "good jobs" from those seeing your results. However I am sure you have heard some of the more negative comments as well. These comments can come in many different forms from back handed compliments to just down right rudeness. I have seen and heard people say things like "you shouldn't lose any more weight because it would be unhealthy." This statement could be true but it was being told to someone who is still well within the obese category. One of my favorites is the "why are you even bothering, you are just going to gain it all back and then some in a year". Their actions can go past comments as well. Tempting you with unhealthy foods then putting you down if you do not accept them.

It is important to not take these comments or actions to heart. If you experience crabs in a bucket scenarios then you know that you are succeeding! Not everyone will be happy for you, some people are so set in their ways and accepted their fate as being overweight and obese that seeing anyone escape that fate is a threat to how they perceive the world. Keep your head held high and stick to what you are doing. The only opinion on your weight loss that matters is yours; just take any criticism as just another obstacle you need to overcome along the way!

135

Join a Fitness or Weight Loss Group

The last section was a little dark but I think it was important for you to be aware that people put down others success so often that there is a metaphor used to describe it. Knowing what it is could help you to not become discouraged if or when you encounter it! Today we will be covering something that is a little lighter. Joining a weight loss or fitness group, and the benefits that can come along with it!

Think back to the sections we covered on the different popular diet programs out there. One of the ones that I said was very good was the weight watchers, which has a built in group component to it. Being a part of the group has shown to increase your ability to stick to a program and achieve your goals! We have also recently covered information about the benefits of brining your family along for the ride. This is also a form of a support group! But what can you do if you do not have a support group available to you? Simple, you join one!

In the internet age you can find a group of people out there that have the same interests and hobbies that you do. The important thing is to find the right group! One of the places that I recommend people trying first in a website called Reddit. This site has the nickname of being the front page of the internet, because once you are on the site there are thousands of "sub reddits" that are communities with a specific purpose. These subs can be about politics, news, pictures of animals, weight loss, and exercise. Finding the right sub could give you a nice group of people who are going through the same thing as you. Subs like r/loseit, r/bodyweightfitness, r/flexibility and r/1200isplentyish are some subs that I think provide good support structures and opportunities for you to discuss issues you might have been having. They will also provide you with information and links to other places that you might find helpful.

You can also search and find various blogs and chat rooms out there that can provide you with support. The important thing to remember is to research everything! Do not just take random strangers on the internet word for it. People might provide you with information and resources that are not correct or safe! Take everything with a grain of salt and conduct your own research. However you might find that joining a cite that could give you support is something that you need to keep you motivated and a great way for you to expand your knowledge of nutrition, and provide you with different workout ideas! It is just something to consider, the world is full of people going through the same things as you and they might be able to offer some help when you need it the most.

136

Fasting

Fasting is something that has become popular in the last several years as a means of weight loss. There can be various types of fasting that include going several hours to days without food, to fasts that allow liquids like water or juice or very small amounts of low calorie solid foods. The question though like always is; does it work?

Take a moment before going on and think critically about everything that we have learned about weight loss and nutrition. How does the body lose weight? Through a calorie deficit where you burn more energy then you take in. Does the body require a large variety of different nutrients to keep itself running? Yes, we need a balance of different types of nutrients, vitamins and minerals to keep our body systems operating. Looking at fasting now will it work? Yes fasting will result in weight loss. You will be consuming very few or no calories which means that your body will need to draw on its fat reserves to run its systems. If your body is relying on fat reserves for energy then you will lose weight it is that simple. However what is the other end of the equation, or should I say the other 2 ends?

First has to do with the nutrients that we are not getting when we are using fat for energy. Fat is not a catch all that stores all of the nutrients as a whole, so it does not necessarily provide you with a balance of nutrition as it is broken down and used. This means that if you are not eating a balanced diet while your fat stores are being broken down for energy you run the risk of becoming malnourished! Secondly, what do we know happens when we do not eat? We can become lethargic, and not want to move much! This can cause us to miss a workout or slow down throughout the day! Remember back to NEAT, if you do not consume enough food it could trigger something in your body to restrict extra movements!

        Although you might have burned more calories from not eating then you would have during your normal daily routine it is likely that it was not much more than if you were to stick to your diet and exercise plan. Is being hungry, tired, and risking malnourishment really worth it to burn only a few extra calories and possibly set you back on your fitness development? I would say that no, it is not worth it! However there is another form of fasting that is becoming popular, and that is intermittent fasting. This is usually when people do not eat for part of the day. Think of it like skipping lunch and only eating breakfast and dinner. This can be an effective way for you to be able to reduce your calories and not risk becoming malnourished, as long as you are still monitoring your calorie intake for the day. I do not have much of an opinion on intermittent fasting mostly because I think it will come down to personal preference. I personally do not do well missing a meal, other people are completely fine skipping lunch or breakfast. The important thing is that you are following along with your daily calorie intake and getting the correct nutrients. I feel that this is best done through regular eating but it is up to you and what you prefer!

If the ingredient list longer than X ingredients, Don't Eat IT

Today is going to be a nice short read; I going to give you a little break today and tomorrow! Today we are going to very quickly cover a myth that likes to pop up from time to time. The idea that if the list of ingredients is so many ingredients long then you shouldn't eat it. I have heard the number of ingredients you shouldn't go over change and range anywhere from 5 to 20 ingredients. So why does this myth keep persisting?

I think that this myth keeps coming back because it could sound like a good idea. Think about it, when you look at the food labels and the list of ingredients there are some foods that look like they have a never ending list of ingredients. So something that has that many ingredients in it can't be good for you right? Well not exactly. As we have learned there are things that are good for us and there are things that are "bad" for us and things that fall everywhere in between. If what you are eating has all sorts of ingredients in it that doesn't mean that it is bad, those ingredients could be great sources of nutrition. On the other hand those ingredients could also be bad, think of foods that contain a lot of different sugars or Tran's fats!

It is easy to want to fall into this idea that the ingredients list is short so it is good for me, or it can't be that bad. This could lead people into the healthy food paradox where it is ok to over eat as long as it's "good" foods. We of course know now that this is just a lie we tell ourselves to make us feel better about over eating! Keep an eye on what you're eating and if you are getting the right amount of nutrients then you don't have to worry about the ingredients list length!

If you Cannot Pronounce it Don't Eat It

Today is going to follow the same nice short format as yesterdays, a very similar topic as well. Today we will go over the idea that if you cannot pronounce the food that you are going to eat then you should not be eating it! Now yesterday I provided a reason why I felt the myth of ingredient list length was popular, I will attempt to do the same with today's myth.

This myth seems to point to the idea that because you cannot pronounce what it is that you are eating then there is no way that it can be good for you. Not only is this a very flawed way of thinking but it doesn't really hold up to just a little bit of thought. I can pronounce all sorts of food that are bad for me, and I have struggled to pronounce some foods when I was first introduced to them such as quinoa. Yet quinoa is a fantastic food that I have found many uses for in the kitchen, it is a great source of protein and other nutrients. Following the line of thinking from the myth, since I didn't know how to pronounce it when I first saw it I should not have tried it. Now we see how dumb the concept is, but could there be a least a little reason behind it? Possibly and here is my take on it. There can be a lot of chemical names for different foods and food products. These names can be difficult to pronounce and even harder to know what they are. So the line of thinking for the myth could be that if you can't pronounce the chemical name then it is probably not good for you. Let's look at one such name. Sorbitol Maltitol Xylitol Mannitol Calcium Carbonite Soy Lecithin Triglyceride Talc. Sounds like a big long scary thing you shouldn't eat, but in reality it is only chewing gum. Although you do not actually eat chewing gum the chemical name for it makes it sound like something you should avoid altogether.

Now we have circled back to the same concept from yesterday. As long as you are making sure that you are staying in your calorie range and getting the proper amount of nutrients in your daily diet then you do not have to worry about things like the chemical names or if you can pronounce the name correctly. Are you starting to see how bad some of these myths really are? Once you become a little educated on the different areas of nutrition it can become very easy to poke holes in so many nutrition and weight loss myths. Think about some of the myths that you have heard or you believed in the past. Are you able to look at them now and see how wrong they really were?

139

Caffeine

We have covered a lot of information so far in this book. We have covered nutrition, how to estimate your calorie expenditures and specific nutrients/ingredients. One that I have mentioned a few times but have not specifically reviewed yet is Caffeine. What is caffeine, should we consume it, how much is too much?

For most working adults a nice shot of caffeine is a way to get yourself moving in the morning, or get you through that afternoon lull. However is this something that you should be doing? Let's go over some of the information and figure it out. Caffeine is classified as a stimulant drug which speeds up the rate that messages are sent from the brain to the parts of the body. It has also been shown to stimulate the release of dopamine which activates the part of the brain that is responsible for alertness and productivity. There can also be a temporary improvement in your mood since dopamine is known to regulate our moods. These effects have also shown to improve our speed and endurance in workouts, which is why caffeine based pre workout drinks have become so popular. All of this sounds great, you can be more alert, happier, and workout harder when you consume caffeine. Are there any downsides?

Well unfortunately yes, there can be downsides to consuming caffeine. When consumed in large amounts, around 500 milligrams which is about 4 large cups of coffee, caffeine has been shown to cause nervousness, irritability, tremors, insomnia, and irregular heartbeat. Ok, so that doesn't sound to great does it? It is common to hear caffeine labeled as addictive, and for many people they might really feel like they are addicted to the stimulant. Although many will argue that you can be addicted to caffeine, it is more of a dependence on the substance. An addiction is when someone has an uncontrolled or compulsive need to use a substance. Although you might feel you have to have caffeine that doesn't mean you can't go without it! When you become dependent on caffeine you can suffer some withdrawal type symptoms when you go without it for a period of time. Some of these symptoms include headache, drowsiness, irritability or depressed mood, difficulty concentrating, and flue like symptoms.

Like any drug it is possible to over dose on caffeine, leading to some serious issues. Although for many they have built up a tolerance to caffeine over the years and over dosing through standard foods and drink could be very difficult. However there are other products out there that offer caffeine in higher doses such as caffeine pills and powders. Consuming these products by themselves or coupled with other caffeine substances could cause dizziness, headache, fever, vomiting, trouble breathing, confusion, heart beat irregularities, seizers, convulsions, and even death.

This section might seem to be playing both sides of the argument, because it is. Caffeine is something that can cause dependence and a whole list of negative side effects. However there are also positive things it can do such as improve your mood and help you concentrate during work or other tasks. It can also be used to help keep you awake when we are feeling drowsy. This is done through a chemical process in the brain. The brain has receptors that adenosine binds to, and when this binding happens we feel tired and go to sleep. Caffeine will actually bind to these adenosine receptors in the brain and effectively shut them off for a period of time, preventing you from feeling tired. The issue with caffeine is similar to issues with many other substances, you have a daily recommended allowance of caffeine that you should try to stay at or under. The recommendation is to stay under 400 milligrams, which is pretty easy to do unless you are consuming specific foods and drinks in large quantities. Consuming several cups of coffee in the mornings and sodas or energy drinks throughout the day could put you over the daily recommend dose. In the end caffeine is something that you really do not need to worry about as long as you are staying within the daily recommended amount, do not have a heart or other conditions that it could effect and if you are not nursing. Caffeine can be transferred to infants through breastmilk causing caffeine overdose if the mother has consumed a high amount. However even in low amounts you could be causing the child to develop a dependence on it or disrupt their sleep patterns.

If you have not already taken some time to track the amount of caffeine that you are consuming throughout the day, maybe you should. Are you staying at or under 400 milligrams? Are you consuming too much or have you developed a dependency on caffeine? If you have then you can take steps to reduce the amount that you consume, however you will want to do this slowly overtime due to the withdrawal symptoms that you could experience. Start by reducing your total amount of caffeine consumed by 50 milligrams per week. After a couple of weeks you should be down into the recommended range and not suffering from the side effects. Like most things that we consume, in moderation it is not bad for you! When you consume to excess there can be a development of health concerns and issues!

140

Exercise: Pull Ups

Pull ups can be an exercise that you hate or love. For many people they are something that they are not even able to complete a single rep of. However if you find yourself in that boat don't worry you can actually do several things if you want to master the pull up. There are two basic classifications of the pull up but the actions are very similar, both resulting in you lifting your body weight up off the ground until you reach the top of the pull up bar. The two types are the pull up which is completed with your palms facing away from you. This method targets more of your back and lats. The other method is known as the chin up. For the chin up you will place your hands on the bar with your palms facing towards you. Due to the anatomical position of the biceps muscle you will activate more of the biceps in this position along with the back and lats. For this section you can use either method, but I will mostly using the term pull up from here on out.

To complete this exercise you will need a bar that is secured above your head. This could be an actual pull up bar like you find in the gym or it could be a door frame pull up bar that is intended for home use. Once you have the bar you will need to get yourself in position by standing directly under the bar. Reach up and find your handholds using either the pull up or the chin up grip. This grip should be at shoulder width or a few inches wider. Once you have your grip you will lift yourself up by flexing at the elbows and the shoulder joint. This action will cause your elbows to bend and lower down to your sides. You will feel the muscles of your arms, shoulders, back, and core tighten during this exercise. Once you have pulled yourself up to eye level or slightly higher than the bar hold for a second or two then slowly lower yourself back down to the starting position. This is one rep.

If you find yourself in the group of people that are not physically strong enough to do a pull up don't worry, you are in good company. The pull up is a very difficult exercise that engages a lot of muscles and that is why it is both a great exercise to add to your daily routine but also very difficult. There are several things that you can do to build yourself up to being able to complete a pull up! If you go to a gym then you can use a variety of machines such as the lat pull down and the assisted pull up. The lat pull down machine is one that functions basically the same way as a pull up except for you remain seated and the bar is pulled down to you. For this machine you can adjust the weight to be lighter or heavier than your body weight. Using this machine will allow you to apply the principle of progressive overload, building up your strength until you are capable of lifting your own body weight to the bar! One of the other machines that is common in the gym is the assisted pull up machine. This machine will have a stationary pull up bar and either a seat or a pad that you will sit or kneel on. The seat is hooked up to weights that pull it up towards the bar. To use this machine you will set a weight and kneel or sit on the pad. Then you get your hand position and complete the pull up. The weights attached to the pad will provide you will assistance by performing some of the exercise for you. Basically what it does is if you set the machine for 50 pounds then it will lift 50 pounds of your body weight and you will lift the rest of your body weight. Over time as you get stronger you can reduce the amount of weight the machine will lift for you and build towards doing the pull up without any help!

That all sounds great but what if you do not go to the gym? There are still options for you. First you will need a pull up bar, such as one that you put in your door way. Once you have one you can try a few options. First you can attach or loop an exercise band over the bar and sit on the ground below the bar. Treat the exercise band like you would the lat pull down machine. Pull the band down towards you against the resistance of the band and simulate the same action as the pull up. This will help to build up your strength to the point that you can do a pull up or you might find this exercise by itself to be ok to stick with. Another method is to get a chair and place it to the side of the bar. Stand on the chair and get yourself into position on the bar at the top of the exercise. Once you are in position lower yourself down slowly to the bottom, or the usual start of the exercise, focusing on the eccentric portion of the lift. We are always stronger on the eccentric portion of an exercise and although you can't lift yourself up in a pull up it is very likely that you can lower yourself down in a controlled manner. Eccentric contractions build muscle just like the concentric contractions! Try getting yourself in the up position and lowering yourself down slowly, take 5-7 seconds to reach the bottom. Once you are at the bottom let go and climb back up to the top of the bar and repeat. Try doing something like 3 sets of 3-5 reps daily. Once it becomes easier increase the time that it takes to lower yourself down. Try making it take 20 seconds or 30 seconds! Over a period of time you will find that you will become strong enough to perform a standard pull up!

If you are adding pull ups to your list of exercises remember to do so safely! Follow the guidelines of the equipment that you are using and perform the movements in a slow controlled manner just like all of the exercises that we discuss. Focus on your mind muscle connection, you will be able to feel your lats contract and tighten! Who knows by the time you hit your weight loss goal you might be able to perform multiple reps of the pull up!

141

Cryotherapy

Cryotherapy can be known by few different names, some of which you might have heard of. These names include cryotherapy, cryolipolysis, and most commonly cool sculpting. This concept is relatively new but does it work? You might be reading this section and have no idea what I am talking about! For some of you it could be a treatment that you are excited to cover because you are curious about it. In this section we will cover what this procedure is and if it will help you or not.

First up, what is cool sculpting? Basically it is a cosmetic procedure similar to liposuction but not invasive! The process uses cold, hence the "cryo" in the name, to destroy fat cells without damaging the surrounding skin or nerves. A device is placed over the area that you would like to be treated such as the under chin or belly. The device then vacuums to the skin and applies cold to the area. This cold effectively destroys the fat cells under the skin, and after a period of time, usually a few months the cells are absorbed back into the body and are effectively gone. On top of that the side effects seem to be minimal and experienced by very few people!

The procedure does not have any recovery time because it is noninvasive and only uses applied cold to the body. What research we have on the treatment shows that participants usually lose 10 to 25 percent of the fat from the area that is treated over a period of 4 to 6 months. Some research has shown that if light massages are applied to the area following the procedures the results can be improved but the effects topped out for this at 4 months. The process usually takes several treatments and can carry a hefty price tag of anywhere from $900 dollars for a small area to more than $1,500 dollars for larger areas per treatment! For most the price tag puts it out of their reach, and since the procedure is classified as cosmetic your insurance will likely not cover it.

Now the big question, does it actually work? The research has shown that it does in fact work for its intended purpose of destroying fat cells. However that is not exactly the right question to be asking. The real questions that should be asked is does it work long term and will it improve your health. The answer to both of these questions is maybe and dependent on the person. Fat is accumulated through the over consumption of calories, and cool sculpting destroys the fat cells that you currently have. However it does not prevent new ones from taking their place! If you do not change your diet and lifestyle then the cells that are removed will be replaced with new fat cells and you will be right back where you started. The procedure will also not improve underlying conditions that are associated with being overweight or having a poor diet. If you have developed diabetes or other health conditions due to excessive body fat or poor diet cool sculpting will not affect them.

If this is something that you have considered or would like to do in the future, discuss it with your primary care doctor and see if it is right for you. Keep in mind that we do not have a lot of data on the long term effects of the procedure and do not know if it could cause issues later in life. As of now it appears that it could be a less invasive alternative to liposuction with similar results of returning fat if diet and life style are not changed. Cryotherapy is not a miracle cure, it will not make you skinny and allow you to spend the rest of your life eating a poor diet and being sedentary. It might aid you in removing some of the last remaining trouble spot hold outs but it should not be used as your primary method of weight loss. Although the process seems effective it is no replacement for a healthy diet and active lifestyle!

142

Saunas

Saunas have been a staple of health clubs and weight loss for decades, but does sitting in a hot sauna actually do anything? Well yes actually there can be some health benefits however not what you might be hoping for or have been told. Let's take a brief look saunas and their effects on our health and weight.

A sauna is a room that is heated up to somewhere between 150 and 195 degrees Fahrenheit. The rooms can be very dry with little humidity or they can be very wet with a lot of steam. There is no difference between the two when it comes to the effects on your body. A sauna session typically runs for 15 to 30 minutes at a time. There has been some research that shows that saunas could be good for your heart in some conditions. When the body experiences high levels of heat your blood vessels will open and move the blood closer to the skin. This is an attempt by the body to have the blood be cooled by the external temperatures; which in most cases works however in a sauna it is not overly effective. When your blood vessels expand your circulation will improve, having a lowering effect on your blood pressure. Some research has shown that there is a link between regular sauna use and heart health. That being said; those with heart issues like irregular heart beat or heart attack are typically advised to avoid saunas. It can be safe for those with high blood pressure to use saunas but the American Heart Associations does not recommend going from extreme hot and cold due to the possibility it could raise your blood pressure.

Now what about saunas effects on weight loss. The truth is that a sauna could help the number on the scale go down! However this is due to the loss of water you experience through sweating in a sauna. The weight will return as soon as you resume proper hydration levels. Saunas have been shown to increase your heart rate though, and as we know an increase in heart rate means more calories being burnt! But again the amount is so low that it really has no effect on weight loss.

In the end there can be some health benefits to regular sauna use, none that include long term weight loss success though. They can be used more for a social experience and possible heart health, but you should consult your doctor before use.

143

Detox Diets

You need to remove the harmful toxins in your body through special detox remedies and products if you want to lose weight. Or so the claims go. I am sure that you have come across the detox claims at some point during your research or general life. Maybe you have tried them or have known someone who has. I have heard people claim you need to detox your body to lose weight, break your addiction to preservatives, improve your sleep and solves all of your ailments. I have seen juice cleanses and vinegar detox concoctions as well as pills you can buy and even special foot baths that will pull the toxins out of your body through your feet. The question is, are our bodies riddled with toxins and should we remove them? Even if it is not through the use of outside products?

Before we answer the question of if you should or should not try a detox diet you should know that there are legitimate detox programs out there. However these programs are implemented by doctors and are usually reserved for drug and alcohol addictions as well as people who have ingested a form of poison. There are no prescribed over the counter detox methods available to the public. Many of the ones you see in infomercials and other Medias are home remedies or do it yourself programs. Proponents of detox diets and products claim that we collect and build up toxins in our bodies through the food we eat, and the environment around us. Then we need to either follow a strict detox diet or use a detox product to "flush" these toxins from our bodies so that we can prevent disease and other ailments.

As I am sure you won't be surprised to hear these methods and products are quackery. You do not need to apply a specific diet or outside product to remove toxins from your body and detox. The truth is that many of the "diets" out there that promote detox can be very dangerous and leave you malnourished and dehydrated. Humans have been on this planet for thousands of years and during all of that time we have been exposed to the elements and materials that are toxic. Our bodies have a method for dealing with these toxins; one of the main ways is through our liver! The liver will take toxic materials that are in the body and convert them to nontoxic then send them off to be expelled from the body through our normal processes. Yes it is possible for certain substances to build up and cause us issues but a detox diet is not going to help in the removal. If a person is suffering from a buildup of toxins that the natural processes of the body cannot handle then they need to seek out medical attention immediately.

If you are concerned with the toxins found in the food we eat and the environment we live in consult your doctor to see what you best course of action should be. I can promise you he will not direct you to a product or remedy you can find for sale or in a meme on social media.

Reminder on Healthy Eating

Since we covered detox diets in the last section I thought it would be a good time to remind you that healthy eating can have more effects on your body then just helping to control your weight! We know that you can lose weight by cutting calories and as long as you are eating fewer calories than you burn then you will lose weight. It does not matter if those calories are from fast food or celery, a calorie is a calorie.

Where the difference comes into play is the nutrients you receive from those calories. Some calories will provide you with more of what your body needs while others can be what we call empty calories. Empty calories provide you with fuel for your body to burn but there are little to no nutrients in them. So although you are fueling your body it is with low quality substances that are not "feeding" your body what it actually needs. In terms of a detox diet we have already covered some things that you can do! Having a daily diet that is rich in high fiber foods will promote colon and digestive health! Think back to the fiber section, it can work as a broom to keep your digestive track clean! This can reduce your risk of cancers and other issues. On the other side of things if you consume a diet high in nutrients, vitamins and minerals then you will reduce your risk of becoming malnourished and keep your body running at peak performance! Reducing your sugar intake will help to keep your blood sugar levels stable and lower your risk of diabetes, and can even reverse some of the of conditions you may have developed!

This was just a brief review to remind you that a healthy diet is not just for weight loss. Typically a poor diet will lead to weight gain; however it is not always a part of it. Having a poor diet even at a healthy weight will still increase your risk of developing chronic conditions! If you have not taken your healthy diet seriously so far I highly recommend that you do!

Weight Loss Surgery

In the modern age we have developed procedures to aid us in weight loss. Millions of people around the world have managed to lose the weight and keep it off through a form of weight loss surgery. The questions though; are they worth it, what are the risks, and should it be something I should consider? Let's take a brief look at some of the types of weight loss surgery's out there and what the results are.

Two of the most popular types of weight loss surgery, also known as bariatric surgery, are gastric band and gastric bypass. One is less invasive than the other but each has different pros and cons. Gastric band involves putting a small adjustable band around the upper part of the stomach to restrict stomach size. The band can be adjusted by injecting or removing the saline in it through a port. The recovery time for this procedure is shorter than other more invasive procedures. The gastric bypass procedure involves converting the upper part of the stomach into a small pouch around the size of an egg. The small intestine is then cut and attached to the pouch, and the other end reattached to the small intestine. This causes food to bypass the majority of the stomach. Both procedures have been shown to give the patient rapid weight loss and allow them to keep the weight off for years to follow. The gastric bypass is heavily invasive and could take a long time to recover from and is permeant, whereas the gastric band can be removed.

I want you to think for a moment about what the weight loss surgeries are actually doing. Why are they successful? The procedures are a method to force a person to restrict the amount of food they consume. This means that calories in vs calories out is still a play here. Weight loss surgery is just a way to make sure that this happens. So why might someone go through the pain, recovery, and high risk of weight loss surgery if it is just the same thing as running a calorie deficit? Typically people opt for the weight loss surgery if they have a BMI of 40 or higher. In cases of extreme obesity people might have difficulty reducing their feelings of hunger even following weight loss. This can be due to a variety of issues include extended stomachs or nerve issues. Restricting the size of the stomach through surgery could help with this issue.

Any surgeries performed on an obese patient carry a higher risk of complication, and weight loss surgery is no exception. It can be a dangerous procedure and most doctors will advise you to try other weight loss options like diet and exercise first. If you feel that you are in need of a weight loss surgery you should thoroughly do your research and discuss all of your options with your primary care doctor. Keep in mind that returning to old dietary habits after surgery can cause major complications; you will still need to make a life style change even after the surgery.

Quality over Quantity

We have spoken several times about the need to focus on quality over quantity when it comes to exercise. All movements burn calories, we have learned about that through section like the one on NEAT. However some movements and activities can burn more calories or workout more of the body than others. That being said just because one exercise burns a higher amount of calories does not mean that it is a good one for you.

Remember the purpose of this book is to teach you about health and wellness so that you can make your own choices and fit it to your lifestyle. I am not here to prescribe you a set of exercises or food you have to eat in order to lose weight. The foods you eat are up to you and the exercise you engage in is decided by you. It is important to do your own research and find exercises that help you reach your goal. That being said depending on your goals you might want to consider selecting exercises that are a little more difficult and give a you better quality workout and burn more calories in a shorter amount of time. Let's look at an example of this. Walking at a slow pace, let's say 3 mph, you will cover a mile in 20 minutes. Depending on your weight you could burn around 100 calories. Now if you were to take the same time frame of 20 minutes and jump rope you could burn over 200 calories! In the end jumping rope could provide double the calories burnt in the same time frame! The quality of the exercise is higher, but so is the difficulty. This is a choice that you have to make when trying to fit exercise into a tight schedule. Do you go for the exercise with higher difficulty and higher calorie burn or the lower difficulty and lower calorie burned. It is up to you, your ability and your goals!

There is another part to the quality vs quantity argument, and it is the more important part. That is performing the exercises correctly! We are going to use the old example of curling a dumbbell. If you are curling the weight and following the guidelines of slow control contraction with a pause at the peak and a slow controlled eccentric contraction as you lower the weight you might not be able to perform as many reps as if you were to lift the weight quickly. Lifting the weight quickly can cause you to miss out on the benefits of the mind muscle connection and parts of the workout like the eccentric phase! You might also use momentum to lift the weight resulting in a reduction of work during the concentric phase. In the end you might have done more reps with sloppy form but the quality and results will not be the same as if you were to focus on doing the exercise correctly and with good form.

In the end it comes down to if you are doing the exercise you might as well do it right. Focusing on quality will give you better results and reduce your risk of injury! Just trying to get in as many reps as you can doesn't mean that you are going to get better result; it might just mean that you are wasting your time!

147

Probiotics

Probiotics are a thing that we hear about all the time in commercials and other Medias but if I was to ask you right now what does a probiotic do. Would you be able to give me a clear answer? Think about this for a few moments. Did you come up with answer? Let me guess it involves something you heard from a yogurt commercial about how they help you to stay or become regular? Regardless of what answer you might have formulated we are going to briefly talk about what a probiotic is and should you add it to your diet.

First up, a probiotic is a blanket term we use to describe the "good" bacteria that is found in our digestive track. This good gut bacteria helps to digest foods, maintain digestive health and support the immune system. When an imbalance in our gut bacteria occurs it can lead to discomfort and diarrhea. Adding probiotics can help restore your gut bacteria to a more optimal level. It has also been shown that adding probiotics to you diet could help reduce symptoms of acute issues like gas, constipation and bloating. You can find probiotics in the foods we eat like plain or Greek yogurt and fermented vegetables like pickles and sauerkraut. There are also over the counter products that come in drinks, pills and powders that you can use to supplement your diet.

It all sounds so good but there has to be a little bad right? Yes, there can be some things that you should watch out for. First know that the research on probiotics is a little thin so we are not really sure on all of the benefits or risks of adding to many probiotics to the body. The other risk comes in a form that we have already discussed. Probiotics are considered a supplement. Do you remember what that means? It means that they are not regulated by the FDA! So the probiotic supplements might not contain high quality ingredients or even the probiotics that are featured on the label! You just cannot be sure about what it is that you are consuming!

If you feel that probiotics are something that you think you might need more of you can try consuming foods that have higher amounts of probiotics in them such as yogurts or pickles. However it is advised that you consult with your doctor to know if you are in need of probiotics or if increasing your consumption of them could have unwanted side effects with your health!

148

Antioxidants

I am going to start today's section off the same way that I did for the last section, with a question. What is an antioxidant? Did some fruit juice commercial pop up in your head that touted the benefits of antioxidants and their effects on free radicals? If that is what you thought of I want to ask you another question. What is a free radical? You might not be sure what a free radical is but it doesn't sound good and you better hurry up and go buy that fruit juice to fight back against them. Well that might be what the juice company would like me to tell you, but I think I will just stick to the facts.

To answer the first question I am going start by answering the second question. What is a free radical? Well to be honest free radicals sound pretty scary when you look at them on paper. They are chemicals that have an appetite for electrons, and will steal them from any nearby substance that they can. Remember back in chemistry class, you would have learned that when a chemical loses or gains an electron their properties can change. In our bodies when a free radical takes an electron from something it can change the chemical makeup of that cell and alter its DNA. They are even able to make our bad cholesterol more likely to get stuck in our arteries!

This is where antioxidants come to the rescue! Antioxidant is a blanket term that covers possibly thousands of substances! What they do is give up electrons to these free radicals preventing them from taking the electrons from us. How heroic of them! Since free radicals seem so dangerous you should probably start buying the different products that contain antioxidants, right? Well yes and no. Antioxidants are not interchangeable so one type is not going to work for every situation and you likely do not need to do anything extra than eat a balanced diet to get all of the antioxidants that you need. Like I had said free radicals sound like a terrifying thing when you look at them on paper but it reality our bodies have been fighting them off since humans came into existence. Some of the more popular antioxidants out there are things like vitamin C and E as well as beta carotene. Sound familiar, well they should! These are already in the foods that you eat. So it is unlikely that you will need to go out and purchase a product to increase you antioxidants because they are already in our regular foods!

As far as products are concerned antioxidants are more of a marketing ploy that allows them to attach claims like the product can help to prevent heart disease, cancer, memory loss and all sorts of other issues. The research has shown that antioxidants can help in these areas but most of the time the products stretch and distort what the results of the studies actually state. In the end if you want to purchase food products that claim to hold antioxidants in them then more power to you. For the average person if you just consume a healthy balanced diet rich in fruits and vegetables then you will have nothing to worry about.

149

Bored Eating

Let's face it eating when we are bored is something that we are all guilty of. One minute you are sitting there watch TV and the next thing you know you are halfway through a bag of chips and there is no sign that you are going to slow down. Today is going to be a short section that looks briefly at bored eating and a little saying you can tell yourself that might help prevent it.

People eat when they are bored for different reasons; just simply being bored is a big reason too! Eating is something to do, even if you are not hungry. You might have seen a commercial on TV about a food product and it made you crave it, or maybe something reminded you about that ice cream that is in the freezer. What you need to be able to do when you are about to eat for no other reason other than you are bored is be honest with yourself. Ask yourself do you want to eat just because you are bored or are you really hungry. That is easier said than done I know. Even the knowledge that you are only going to eat because you are bored might not be enough to prevent it! When you catch yourself about to boredom eat, stop and go look for something to do. It can be a chore or a hobby, anything that isn't eating. This could stop you from consuming those extra calories that you really don't need. Now what if you think you might be hungry but it could just be the boredom talking? Well ask yourself are you hungry enough to eat an apple? If you think you are hungry but not hungry enough to eat an apple then simply put, you are not hungry!

Eating when you are bored is something that happens and it can set your weight loss back a day or more. The important thing is to not let it happen too often. When you notice that you are bored eating or wanting to, take control and prevent it. Go do something else productive or eat an apple. Apples are low in calories and could help to prevent you from over eating higher calorie junk foods! This same strategy can be applied to stress eating as well!

Entering the Last Month

You have come such a long way and this book is nearly completed! Think back to the day you read section 1 and look at how far you have come. By now you have taken control over your diet and have slowly implemented long lasting lifestyle changes that will set you up to maintain your weight loss for years to come! If by this time you have met your weight loss goal congratulations! If you haven't got there yet keep on following what you have learned in this book and you will get there. Take today to reassess your TDEE and get an accurate daily calorie count going forward.

In this final month we are going to continue to go over some health topics as well as information that you can use to continue to apply to your life long after you reach the last page! Keep up the great work and continue to apply what you have learned. If you are not finding success or have stalled out a little review the section on plateaus and reassess your calorie intake for the day. Check to make sure that you are accurately recording your calorie intake and your portion sizes.

Check to make sure that you are still on track to meet your goals! Remember monitoring your progress to your goal and breaking your larger goals down into smaller milestone goals is a great way to stay motivated. Take today and congratulate yourself on your progress. Losing weight is an easy concept but can be difficult in practice! What you have accomplished so far is amazing.

Calorie Tip: Wraps Vs Bread

So you are out getting lunch or making lunch at home, you turn to the always favorable sandwich. With your new healthier diet you decide to opt for the wrap instead of your usual two slices of bread. Wraps are the healthier choice right? Well not exactly!

Wraps can be a good alternative to certain breads and might help reduce your calorie count when compared to just breads. However for the most part they are similar in calorie count but wraps are more likely to contain higher levels of sodium and Tran's fats. Both of which are things that we should try to reduce in our diets. This means that a wrap may or may not be a healthier choice when it comes to the wrap vs bread argument! If you are someone who enjoys eating wraps over the standard two slices of bread sandwich then do your research. Read the food labels of the bread you buy and the wraps you purchase. Opt for the ones that contain whole grain and no hydrogenated oils, which if you recall is just another name for Tran's fats. You might find that your wraps are not the best choice for you after all! Or you might be able to find an option that is "close enough".

There has to be more to this section then just compare the food labels between wraps and bread, right? Well yeah. When it comes to wraps vs bread, what goes inside them is arguably more important than which one you decide on. Wraps can be very large; some of the wrap options out there are the size of a dinner plate! This is where the negatives for wraps can really take off. If you are making a sandwich on standard bread then you do not have a great deal of space to put the contents of your sandwich on. If you are using a wrap the size of a dinner plate then you are more likely to add more ingredients and condiments. More ingredients equals more calories.

In the end if you are eating wraps because you believe they are healthier than a standard sandwich then make sure that you are not over eating because of the size of the wrap! There are things you can do however! The simplest one is to just use smaller wraps. If you are not able to put as much stuff in them then you will not be over eating! Make sure that you are comparing the nutritional information and make the best choices for you! Don't fall for the "it is the healthier choice" idea without checking into it yourself!

Happiness

Today will be a short section on happiness and you. We have learned that exercise can release endorphins in our brains that can improve our moods and make us feel happier. This is a temporary sensation but with regular exercise you could keep the good times rolling so to speak. We have also learned that our food choices can affect our moods and how much energy we have during the day. The amount of energy we have or how well our bodies feel as a result of healthier foods can also contribute to how happy we are.

The problem is that although exercise and a healthy lifestyle in and off itself can improve our moods it might not be enough. If you are becoming more fit and reaching your weight loss goals but still finding yourself unhappy then there could be more to it than your body composition, diet and exercise habits. You need to look deep into yourself and search out what is the root of your unhappiness. If need be consult a close friend or a professional.

If you are not happy in your life then keeping the weight off might be a harder thing for you to accomplish. During this journey we have made action plans on how to improve your health and reach your weight goals. Take the same principles and create an action plan on how to become happier. Find the root cause of it and come up with a strategy to make improvements! A healthier lifestyle includes your mental health too!

Challenge Yourself

We are faced with challenges every day. Some are place upon us through our responsibilities such as work, school, and children. Others are created by us to help improve ourselves. Just picking up this book was a way of challenging yourself. You decided that you wanted to make a change, and you have been making those changes over the last 153 days. The "challenge yourself" concept will be a little different for today's section.

One thing that myself and many other people like to do is challenge ourselves to a physical task to complete. This is very similar to the goals that we create but can differ in many ways. In the past I have challenged myself to doing 100 push-ups every day for a month, or to do 50 pull ups every day for a month. These challenges were a way for me to give myself something to compete for; something to push myself to achieve. I might not be able to complete the challenge early on. Doing 100 push-ups in a day might be a little much at the start. I might have to do 10 sets of 10 reps. Then soon it is 5 sets of 20 reps. Soon I will be at 4 sets of 25 reps, and then 2 sets of 50. By the end of the month I might be able to complete 1 set of 100 reps. This not only increases my muscle strength and endurance, but it also gives me a sense of accomplishment! I set out to do something and by the end of the month not only could I do it but I could do it better than I ever expected!

Try applying this to your physical activity. Maybe you want to push yourself to do 30 crunches every day for a week or a month. Maybe you would like to walk a mile every day and that is the challenge you set. Look for something that you like to do or something that you want to be better at then dedicate a couple weeks or a month to accomplishing it! You might find that you can become highly motivated and competitive with yourself. We have about a month left of readings, if you start today then your first challenge could wrap up at the same time as this book!

Healthy at Every Size

There have been various movements throughout the years that seek to help people be more positive about your body. One of the biggest movements right now is the Healthy at Every Size movement. The idea behind this is for you to accept your body for what it is and that your size does not dictate your health.

Of course being body positive is something that anyone can get behind. You should strive to feel comfortable in your own skin. As we have already discussed just being thin or fit does not mean that you will be happy. The HAES community promotes the idea that you can be healthy and big or healthy and fit and you should be what you are most happy with. The truth is that you can be healthy at every size. However that doesn't mean that you will remain healthy at a bigger size. One of the things I hear often is "my blood work shows that I am fine!" This very well could be true, but blood work is not the only indicator of good health. Over the last 154 days we have gone over all sorts of different risk factors and how you're increasing your percent chance of developing conditions like diabetes and heart disease. Take a male who is 6ft tall 170 pounds at 40 years who has been active for the last 20 years and compare him to a male of equal height and age but is 400 pounds and has been sedentary for the last 20 years. Given all of what we know, who would you place your bet on to contract a chronic illness or disease like diabetes? Yes they could both be healthy but one is at a far greater risk!

Body acceptance is a great thing but there can be a point where it will have a negative impact on your current health or your future health. One of the issues I have with the HAES community is that the more extreme end of the movement does more than promote body positivity, they promote and glorify obesity. People are able to be healthy when obese but that doesn't mean that it should be promoted as a positive life style. Take care of the body you have now, you only get one. Take steps to reduce your risk factors and you might find that you will be able to accept your body for a much longer time!

155

Cooking Foods Can Add Calories

There have been debates back and forth for years between cooked or raw foods, and which is better for you. This idea is mostly about vegetables since most people would not want to or be advised to consume raw meats or poultry. However there is a case to be made that cooking food increases the calories in that food.

This increase in calories can come down to a couple of causes. The first cause is something that might seem like a no brainer. When we cook foods we rarely cook them without adding ingredients. We add in seasonings, liquids, other foods, all things that typically contain calories. So if you are cooking a roast and the nutritional information is saying that roast will give you 200 calories per serving that is only including the meat. It is not taking into account any seasoning or add in's that you used during cooking. When you are cooking you need to take into account all of the ingredients that you are using and their serving size.

Ok that was the easy one, now for the 2nd way cooking foods can cause more calories. The first way was due to us physically adding other calories to the food; this way is increasing your ability to absorb more of the calories from the food itself. Remember back in prior sections we discussed how you do not absorb 100 percent of the calories in the food you eat. Some calories are burnt in the digestive process and this reduces your net gain of calories for that food. While other calories are just never broken down in digestion and absorbed. These calories will pass through the body and never get used. When we cook food it is like we are starting the digestive process before we ever eat it. Cooking food breaks down some of the cells and nutrients of that food which in turn will allow our digestive systems to break down the food even further.

Basically some of the work is already done for us! So in the end cooked food provides more digestible calories than raw foods.

So it sounds like it might be a good idea for you to eat your veggies raw so that you absorb fewer calories. This could be the case but did you consider all of the factors. If cooking the foods makes it easy for our bodies to digest and absorb calories then that also means that it could make it easier for our bodies to absorb more nutrients as well. As we know our bodies rely on a balance of nutrients and different vitamins and minerals. Cooking our foods can make it easier for our bodies to get what we need to keep our systems going.

Sounds like a double edged sword doesn't it? The cooked food might provide more calories but also provides more nutrients than uncooked foods. In the end I suggest you don't worry about it so much. Remember what I said about trying to get to specific with your diets? All you will do is complicate it too much and make it harder to keep track of then it needs to be. If you like eating raw vegetables then eat raw vegetables. If you like cooked veggies then eat them cooked. It comes down to what you like and what works for you. This book is not about giving you specific foods to eat or not eat or specific workout to do. Understanding that there is a difference between cooked and uncooked but not one that will alter your weight loss by much is important to your understanding of how the body works and maintaining a healthy lifestyle.

156

Injuries Happen

One of the risks of being more active is injury. If you are moving more and participating in activity then you might develop strains, sprains, and other more serious injuries. The problem with these injuries that you might encounter is that they could slow down or stop your weight loss. Your motivation and drive could also be effected by injurie. The physical effects are not the only thing you need to be concerned about when injured, your mental state can also be negatively affected.

If you find yourself getting injured during your weight loss or after you met your goal weight then you will find that it might be difficult to keep going. For many people and possibly for you, being physically active is an important part of your weight loss plan. We take activity level into account when we are finding our TDEE's and figuring out our daily caloric allowance. If you are injured and end up having to sit on the couch or reduce activity for an extended period of time then you need to reassess your TDEE to reflect the amount of exercise you are getting throughout the day. Depending on your injury and your doctor's orders you might be able to make adjustments to your activity level to try to compensate a little. For example if you have a broken arm then you can still walk around. Going for a walk every day is still a way to get exercise. If you have a sprained ankle then maybe getting an exercise band and performing some upper body resistance exercise could be your exercise while you heal up. The important thing is to do what you can, how you can. Staying active even if it is less than you were prior to your injury can help to keep you motivated.

I have had some pretty bad injuries in the past, one of which had me lying on a couch for 7 months. I went from working out an hour or more a day for 6 plus years to laying on the couch watching TV from the time I woke up until it was time for bed. This experience showed me how hard it really can be to start over from square one. My physical endurance was gone, my muscle mass shrank, however I prevented fat accumulation by reducing my daily caloric intake. Starting over is not easy and it can be very hard on your motivation to get back into things. You have been working very hard on becoming more fit as well as losing weight, and if you become injured all of your progress could come to a screeching halt. It is important that you find a way to stay motivated to keep up with your daily calorie goals while injured. Your weight loss might slow down during an injury but if you are monitoring your calorie intake then you will not gain the weight back. When you are cleared to go back to your activity level you will notice that you have lost some or all that you gained through your hard work. Don't be afraid to start over, you made improvements and gains before you can do it again. Thanks to "muscle memory" you can do it again and a little quicker this time around! Don't get discouraged if you have an injury, make an adjustment and get back to reaching your goal as soon as you are able to.

157

Muscle Memory

Muscle memory is something that I mentioned in the last section, but what is it? The way I used it, it made it seem like out muscles will "remember" our old activity level and adjust to it more quickly than when we were first starting out. This is one of the common ideas when it comes to muscle memory. The other is that our muscles will eventually remember our repetitive movements and we will be able to perform them without much or any conscious thought. Think of an athlete like a pole vaulter, when they take off from the ground and catapult themselves into the air they are performing a series of timed movements and adjustments to make it all happen. They need to press out with their lower arm to bend the pole vault pole then drive their non-jumping knee followed by swinging the jumping leg through while collapsing the lower arm by bending at the elbow to get upside down on the pole. After that they have to row with their arms at the peak of the poles force while unbending to throw themselves off of the pole to get the most height. This is all done in about 2 seconds and is possible because of muscle memory. However this is not the type of muscle memory that we will be covering in this section.

When we talk about muscle memory as it pertains to gaining muscle strength through exercise we are talking about the ability of the body to regain lost muscle more quickly the 2nd time around. We know how the body increases muscle mass already. The body adapts to the stress of exercise by building up our muscles overtime to meet that stress. When we are no longer using our muscles against that stress then the body will reduce the size of the muscles. This is called atrophy and is a natural process of the body. So if you are lifting weights and after a year you have made some great gains in muscle strength and size then you stop for 6 months your muscles will reduce in size and strength. However if you were to return to lifting weights you might have to start out where you did the first time but this time around you will gain in muscle size and strength much faster. Why does this happen?

As we build muscle through exercise our muscles will increase the number of nuclei in our muscle fibers. These nuclei aid in protein synthesis which is part of the muscle building process. Once the nuclei are constructed in our muscle fiber they remain there long after we stop exercising and our muscles atrophy. So when we return to lifting weights or exercising our bodies do not have to build these nuclei again to aid in protein synthesis, the building blocks are already in place. Because our bodies do not need to go through the nuclei building process again it can focus on building the muscle back up resulting in faster muscle gains then the first time around.

Currently we do not know how long the nuclei will remain in the muscle fiber following atrophy. It could be a long period of time like several years or a short period of time of several months. It could also be different for each person. However what this means for you is that if you take time off from your exercising it might feel like you are starting over from scratch but in reality you already have the ground work laid and you will get back in shape much faster than you originally did!

158

Diuretics

A diuretic is probably a term that you have heard before. You might even take some as they are a popular medication to help reduce blood pressure. What is it that Diuretics actually do? Basically they help the body to remove sodium and water from the blood stream. This causes the volume of blood in our bodies to go down resulting in lower blood pressure. You might be asking yourself; why are we covering diuretics in this book if it is a blood pressure medication?

Simply put, diuretics have found their way into the weight loss supplement world! If you think about it, why might a diuretic be used for weight loss? Often weight loss pills or supplements will make claims that you can lose 10 pounds in the first week. These claims are usually true but the weight you lose is not body fat it is water weight. Many weight loss supplements use diuretics so that you will quickly reduce the amount of water weight in your body and keep it off while you are on the product. This follows the same concept as saunas; weight loss through loss of fluid is not fat loss. As soon as you return to proper hydration levels your scale will return to showing your higher weight. However with weight loss products that use diuretics you will find that as long as you keep taking them you will keep the water weight off. As soon as you stop taking them you will gain the water weight back, and quickly. This rapid return of weight might trick some people into thinking that they need the product in order to keep the weight off and just like that a repeat customer is born!

There can be some issues when you are consuming diuretics. First you could experience mineral loss through the frequent urination and might experience potassium loss leading to muscle cramps. Continued use could lead to low sodium in your blood, dehydration, joint disorders, headaches and dizziness. If you are already on blood pressure medication do not begin taking weight loss supplements before discussing it with your doctor.

Although I do not recommend turning to over the counter weight loss supplements because the side effects can be vast. The FDA does not regulate supplements so there is no check of if the ingredient lists are correct or if their claims are factual. If you are considering taking a weight loss pill consult with your doctor, they will be able to go over your best options. If you were considering using weight loss supplements or have in the past check for the use of diuretics. The results you see might just be nothing more than water weight. You could very well be just flushing your money down the toilet!

159

Eating at the Holidays

In the United States one of the things that we as Americans love to do during the holidays is eat! We eat pie and turkey during Thanksgiving; we eat cookies during Christmas, ham during Easter and so on. It is so easy for people to over eat during the holiday. In fact almost everyone does! I know I am certainly guilty of it. Should you be concerned about the amount that you eat during the holidays or is the one day of over eating ok?

Over eating a single day here and there is not going to cause you to suddenly gain all of your weight back. It could set you back several days or a week when it comes to your calorie deficit but you're not going to find yourself 15 pounds heavier because you over did it a little on Thanksgiving. Truth is that you very well could gain a pound or more of fat depending on what you ate and how much you ate of it. At this point you know how calories work! However for many of us the holidays are a time of good times with friends and family and good food. Splurging a little is ok. However you need to keep in mind that there are 6 major holidays in the United States that we celebrate with high calorie foods. There is Christmas, New Years, Easter, Independence Day, Halloween, and Thanksgiving. 6 major holidays works out to an average of 1 major holiday every other month. So over eating every other month is really not that bad.

There are things that you can do to try and mitigate the amount that you will gain during the holidays! First you need to be cautious of the food you eat leading up to the holidays. There are cookies everywhere during the Christmas season and you could end up wrecking your diets for the whole month instead of just one day! Halloween candy goes on sale well before October even rolls around. It is easy to pick up a bag or two of candy early with the intention of using it for the trick r' treaters only to pick at it until you have eaten it all. If you are cheating on your healthier diets during the holiday seasons you could be causing yourself to lose out on up to 6 months of progress! What you eat between the holidays is more important than what you eat on the Holiday.

Monitor yourself closely during the holiday seasons; they will test your will power. You can prepare for the holiday feast by cutting a few extra calories for the week leading up to the celebration. Try cutting out an extra 50 calories a day for the week before this will give you 350 calories to spare on the day of. You could also try doubling that and cut 100 extra calories a day for the week before. This would give you 700 calories of extra room so that you do not set yourself back as far! You of course could always eat less at the holidays as well. You can still over indulge in the high calorie foods but eat one piece of pumpkin pie instead of 2. Only drink that one beer at the 4th of July picnic instead of 3. Self-control and prepping between the holidays takes a little effort but ask yourself is pushing your weight loss goal back so you can have that extra piece of pie really worth it?

160

How to Conduct Your Own Research

I have recommended that you complete your own research several times throughout this book, but what does it actually mean and how do you do it? Simply using an internet search engine and picking the top result doesn't always cut it. The way you worded your search could be off or the top results could be paying to show up at the top. There are countless resources out there, some are good, some are bad, and some are flat out wrong. How do you know what to trust?

First you start with a specific question, specific questions get specific answers. Searching how to lose weight on the internet returned almost 1 billion results! There are several "how to lose 10 pounds in 10 days" and "Follow these 20 tips to easy weight loss" articles. Some of the tips and articles get some of the information correct and some of the information wrong, others are just plain quackery. Redefining my search to a more specific question of "how to lose weight through calorie counting" lowered my search results total to 8 million. That is an enormous drop! The results were more informative and specific to what information I was looking for.

Next you need to develop background information on the topic of your question. This can include doing things like familiarizing yourself with the terminology of the subject. If I was to search a specific question about rebuilding an engine for a 1994 ford tempo but I didn't know the first thing about cars then I would likely not understand the information that I was reading. If I am not able to understand what it is that I am reading then there is no point to reading it. Take the time to look into the information that you want and know how to understand it not just read it.

The next step is to gather more information. So you have researched the information you want, and you searched your specific question and now you are reading articles about it. Do not just read one single article, branch out and read other articles about the topic. Try to collaborate the information over several sources. The more sources that say the same information the more likely it is to be correct. Then try including peer reviewed academic articles on the subject. Search engines like Google let you specifically search for these kinds of articles. Academic journals tend to be written more like text books and can be hard to decipher if you have no prior knowledge. However now that you have researched the information thoroughly then you should be able to check what the current research is saying. Try reading the Abstract or the Conclusion to find the results.

Finally you need to evaluate the quality of your sources. If you are reading certain information you found on some ones blog that contradicts what your other sources like academic journals are saying then you might not want to trust the blog as an accurate source. A good way to test if the information is correct is to read arguments for and against the information that you have found. For example if you research a weight loss product such as the fat fighter pills we discussed in an earlier section then you might see all sorts of positive reviews and glowing testimonials on their website. There might even be research present to try to show the validity of the products claims. The pills must work right because they show research and testimonials showing how good they are, right? Researching the counter arguments is a great way to find "holes" in the claims or research that they showed. Remember back to the apple cider vinegar section where the research showed that those who took the apple cider vinegar lost more weight than those who didn't? Those results might make you believe that consuming it would boost your weight loss even if only a little. Then I showed you another study that found that participants lost weight because they were too nauseous to eat following the consumption of the apple cider vinegar. If you did not do additional research you might have found out about the nausea the hard way!

In the end the more research you do the better informed you will be. Look into the credentials of who is writing the information, are they a person who is not certified in the field and is just writing a blog or are they an exercise physiologist who conducted the research. I like to follow a saying I heard in college. If you cannot argue both sides of the point then you do not know enough about the subject to hold a solid opinion. This means know the points for and against something so that you can make an educated evaluation and decision. Thoroughly researching a subject properly can lead you to being better informed and better prepared for whatever it is that you are trying to accomplish!

161

Cholesterol

Cholesterol is a substance found in our bodies and the foods that we eat; it is something that our bodies need in order to function properly. There are two types of cholesterol that get all of the attention, the first is HDL or High Density Lipoprotein and the second is LDL; or Low Density Lipoprotein. One is known as the good cholesterol while the other is the bad, but do you know which one is which? Do you know why one is bad and the other isn't, or does your knowledge of it end at one is bad?

To begin, cholesterol is a waxy substance found in our cells that is similar to fat. It is a substance that we use to help make hormones, vitamin D, and digestive substances. Our body is actually capable of creating all of the cholesterol that we need! However we do get some from the foods that we consume. If your body has too much in its blood stream then you run a higher risk of developing artery clogging plaque. When plaque builds up in your arteries you can develop coronary artery disease which is when your arteries become narrow or even fully blocked! From the sounds of things we don't want too much of either good or bad cholesterol to build up in our bodies, do we?

LDL is not all bad; our bodies still use it for various functions. When we start to develop higher levels of it within our blood is when we need to start to worry about it. As I mention it can cause your arteries to clog up or even close. This could lead to a heart attack or stroke as well as death. Where HDL, good cholesterol, differs is in its function within the body. HDL will actually carry cholesterol from different parts of your body back to your liver where it will be removed from your body. So having higher levels of HDL could mean that your body is more efficient at removing unneeded cholesterol from the body.

There are several factors associated with having bad cholesterol; some of us just were unlucky enough to have it run in our families while others develop it through our life choices. The most common contributor to high LDL is unhealthy dietary habits. Those of you who had high cholesterol prior to the start of this book, has changing your diet to a healthier one helped lower your LDL? Over time improvements in diet can help to lower your levels of LDL and improve your levels of HDL. What are some of the foods you need to watch out for that can increase your risk of high cholesterol? Eating the bad fats such as saturated fats found in some meats and dairy products. Baked goods that contain saturated and Tran's fats and deep fried foods can also lead to high LDL.

Your activity level can have great effects on your levels of HDL, the good cholesterol! The more sedentary you are the lower your HDL level can become. Remember the HDL helps to clean up cholesterol throughout the body. Lowering your HDL could increase your levels of LDL! What we eat and how much activity we get seems to be the best indicator of cholesterol problems or lack thereof. If you are someone with cholesterol problems following the guidelines in this book could help lower your LDL. Try reducing your consumption of red meats and fried foods, even if they are fitting into your daily calorie budget. Seek out advice from your doctor if you have or feel you have high cholesterol, they can advise you of your options.

162

Body Weight Squats

Have you ever heard someone tell you to lift with your legs not your back, only to immediately lift whatever it was with your back? Most people probably have. On the same line of thinking have you ever heard that squats are one of the best exercises you can do? I am sure that is something that you have also heard. When it comes to the squat it is a fantastic exercise that will work a large amount of muscles and can be used in your daily life to make tasks easier. That is why the squat is classified as a fundamental movement by the American Council on Exercise. When you are able to perform the squat correctly you will be able to use it to help make your life easier and reduce your risk of back injury.

When you squat down to pick something up whether heavy or light you will reduce the amount of pressure that is put on your back and neck. When you squat with good form you are keeping your spine in a straight natural position and you are not extending your upper body out past your center of gravity. Keeping your spine in the neutral position is often referred to as "keeping your spine in line". When we do this it prevents us from bending at the waist and extending our upper body out. When we extend our upper body out by bending at the waist we are putting strain on the lower back. This strain is caused by the fact that our upper body weighs a lot and the further we bend over at the waist the further things like our head get from the center of the body. The further out they go the more weight and strain is placed on the lower back. This can lead to back pain and strains. The squat is a way to lower yourself down by bending at the knees and some of the waist. Performing this exercise will activate the glutes, quads, core, and hamstrings to an extent. It hits all of the major muscles of the lower body. The glutes (butt) however, perform most of the work.

Performing the squat is actually very simple. First you will need to stand with your feet about shoulder width apart, point your toes slightly outward. Most people like to put their hands together and place them on their heads or on their hips, hand placement can be anywhere you feel comfortable. Next you will begin to lower yourself towards the ground by bending at the knees. As you begin to lower you will bend slightly at the waist allowing your head and shoulders to remain over your center of gravity. Once you have reached a point where your upper legs are parallel with the ground you may stop. In this parallel position your feet should be flat on the ground, your knees should not be further than your toes and your waist should be at about a 45 degree angle from your upper leg. When your waist is bent at this angle you should feel you butt being pushed out slightly and your back should be in straight line. You may now finish the squat by returning to the starting position. Begin to press up by pushing through your heels and straightening your legs and waist. Once at the top you have completed 1 repetition.

Try adding the body weight squat to your daily routine. Take a couple minutes every day and do 3 sets of 10 repetitions. If you cannot lower yourself down to parallel go as far as you can. Overtime work on going further and further down. If Parallel begins to get to easy try going lower or adding weight to the squat. You might even shape up your back side!

163

Things Food Products Will Claim

Have you ever looked around at the different boxes and packages of food at the grocery store? If you have you will notice that there are all sorts of claims plastered all over them. Some of them suggest that there is "no fat" while others say "heart health" or "no added sugar". Are these claims true? Are they stretched a little? How much should we really believe?

By now you are aware that some products use exaggerated claims or promote certain aspects of their product in order to get you to purchase them. Someone might be deciding between two very similar products but one had "No Tran's Fats" plastered right on the box. You will likely buy the one that says no Tran's fats simply because you know that Tran's fats are not good and the other product doesn't specifically say that it doesn't contain Tran's fats. We have briefly gone over this concept in the section on fruit juices. One product might say "no added sugar" but that doesn't mean that it has no sugar or that it has any less sugar than the other similar products.

Some claims could be good, such as the "source of" type claims. You might see these claims on products such as dairy claiming "a good source of calcium" or in the produce section "a good source of vitamin C". Although these claims could technically be correct it doesn't mean that they are the best source of vitamin C or calcium. Any product that has any vitamins or minerals in it could technically put on its box that it is a source of that vitamin or mineral. That doesn't mean that it is still the best source or the best product for your needs. One of the other common claims is the "risk factor" claim. "This product reduces your risk of..." followed by some sort of ailment like heart disease or osteoporosis. Following the results of some of those studies I mention in the Apple Cider Vinegar section, that product could put on their label that it "could reduce your risk of obesity". Technically the research did show weight loss as a result of consuming it; it was just because it made them too sick to eat! So those claims might not always be wrong, but that doesn't mean they are correct either!

It will always be best to read the information for yourself. Don't let what some advertiser put on the packaging dictate which products you buy. A product with no added sugar could still be high in sugar. Check your nutritional labels and see what is contained in each product. This does not mean that the claims on the box are always false or misleading. Often times you might find that the "good source of calcium" type claims are in fact a good source of calcium. However that doesn't mean that the other product couldn't offer similar amounts of calcium but with fewer calories! Check your labels and know what it is that you are purchasing. Don't fall for every claim or trick on the product box. Starting your dietary choices in the grocery store means that you are setting yourself up for success at home! Bring home the best foods to meet your dietary needs so that you are not leaving any room for guessing. If you don't think you should be eating it then simply don't buy it. You cannot eat junk food you never brought home!

164

Pre-Workout

If you have been around the fitness community at all then you likely have heard about Pre-Workout supplements. These supplements are typically a powder that you mix with water and drink 15 to 20 minutes before you begin your workouts. They claim to boost your energy levels, performance, and concentration. All of those things sound like they will be a perfect addition to give you the edge in your workout. Is a pre-workout something that you should be adding to your routine?

Pre-Workouts typically advertise a few similar ingredients within their products. First you will see vitamins being promoted as the cause of the boost in energy and performance. In reality the vitamins are typically not found to have much of or any actual effect on your energy level or performance. So where does the energy come from? I am sure that you already know or have guessed the answer to that question. Caffeine. Yes, caffeine is one of the major ingredients in pre-workout supplements and is usually the ingredient responsible for your boost in energy. As we have learned caffeine is not inherently bad, and when taken in moderation there are energy and performance boosting properties to it. Where you need to be cautious is in the amount of caffeine! A typical pre-workout contains the same amount of caffeine as 4 cups of coffee! That can be similar to some larger energy drinks that we have already covered. This is a very large dose of caffeine that is ingested in a very short amount of time and can cause your heart to race or your heart to have irregular beats.

One of the side effects that you might notice from taking a pre-workout supplement is itchy skin and tingling in your hands feet and face. This can be an unpleasant feeling but it is only temporary. The sensation is caused by two common ingredients found the supplements. The first one is an amino acid known as Beta-alanine. This amino acid is nonessential because our bodies can create it from other amino acids; however its intended use in a pre-workout is to reduce your muscle fatigue during a high intensity workout. The other culprit of the itchy feeling is Niacin, or vitamin B3 that your body uses for energy metabolism.

The real questions are do they work and are they safe. Yes the pre-workouts can work and help give you a boost to get you through your workouts. The same results however can probably be found by drinking a cup of coffee before you work out; meaning that yes they can work but are not needed. Now is it safe? It can be. When you follow the instructions on the label and ensure that you are remaining in your nutritional daily values then yes you could say they are safe. With that being said consult your doctor before you would decide to try one. Your doctor can advise you on if you personally will be ok taking the supplement.

165

BCAA

Continuing with our theme of workout supplements we are going to discuss BCAA's today. BCAA or "branch chain amino acid" supplements are becoming very popular in the fitness community lately, but are they worth the time or money? What we have learned so far tells us that amino acids are the building blocks of muscles and that we have essential amino acids; meaning we cannot produce them ourselves and non-essential amino acids meaning that we can create them from other sources. In your typical BCAA complement you will find 3 essential amino acids Isoleucine, leucine, and valine.

Since the amino acids found in the BCAA supplements are essential amino acids that means that our bodies have to get them from an outside source. It boils down to the supplement can provide something that you will need. Some of the claims around BCAA's are that they will aid with protein synthesis and your recovery following a workout. Are these claims true however? Well yes and no. Yes the amino acids found in the BCAA supplements are essential they are not complete and will not give you results on their own. You will still need to consume complete forms of protein to get their benefits. Furthermore many of the supplements will contain artificial sweeteners and other manufactured ingredients to add taste or color to the product. We have also learned and repeated several times that a supplement is not regulated by the FDA so the nutritional label of the supplement could be misleading.

In the end a BCAA supplement could help you to get the essential amino acids you need for your body to build muscle following a workout. However, you will find that many of the claims from the product are exaggerated. You will not see improved results from the supplement alone and will still need to make up for the supplements short comings in your normal diet. When it really comes down to it your diet is the best pre-workout and post workout "supplement" you can take. Maintaining a balanced diet where you are achieving your daily nutritional goals will render all of the supplements useless. If you feel that you need to increase your protein consumption or would like to try a BCAA supplement for yourself remember to do your own research on the product. Find out what is in the supplement and if your body is really in need of what is being provided by the product. It is very likely with you healthy diet that you are getting all of the nutrients that you need and adding in any additional protein or amino acids will get filtered through your bodies systems and removed through excrement. If you still believe that you need or want to try the supplement, discuss it you're your doctor to be sure that it is the right choice for your health and well-being!

Cravings

Cravings are something that everyone deals with. Sometimes you are just hungry for some particular type of food whether that is salty or sweet or maybe even savory. The point is that you just want it! However have you begun to notice that your cravings for certain types of foods decrease? Are your cravings starting to change? Similar to the habits that we have been working on changing for the last 166 days, your cravings will eventually change as well

Remember back to what we learned in the artificial sweetener section, one of the issues that artificial sweeteners can cause is an increase in a person's craving for sweet foods! What does this tell us? Our cravings can be influenced by our own diets. When we consume foods that contain simple carbs our blood sugar can spike and for some people these simple carbs can give a euphoric feeling for their brain not unlike a drug. This is because the simple carbs might trigger pleasure centers in our brain! This feeling can cause the brain to want it more once the feeling subsides causing you to crave more simple carbs. What else do we know about simple carbs? They are digested quickly and do not provide you with the feeling of being full for a long time. Consuming a regular diet of simple carbs could be setting you up to not only eat more often due to the early return of hunger feelings but also cause you to crave the same type of foods in order to get that feeling back. Research has shown us that diets high in simple carbs can actually be addictive or cause dependence!

This addiction to the food that you eat could lead to some very intense cravings that are hard to overcome! Think back to your dietary habits prior to starting this book. Did you find yourself having cravings for the type of foods that contain simple carbs or the "junk foods"? Were you always giving in and eating something even though you knew you shouldn't but you were craving it? For many this is the case, they are chasing the good feelings that became associated with the foods they ate. This makes weight loss and weight management harder for many. However you have been working on controlling your diet for over 5 months now! Have you begun to notice that your cravings for certain foods have gone down? Are you beginning to associate those "good feelings" with the healthier more complex food choices? Over time our bodies are able to break the addiction that we feel with certain foods. That is not to say that you won't still have cravings for a certain food or flavor from time to time, but you should be feeling them less and less.

Keep in mind that it is not the end of the world if you give into a bad food craving! We have covered topics similar to this in the past. Cutting out all of the food you love will only make you want it more and overindulge in that food. Feeding your cravings from time to time can actually help you stay on track, as long as you do not make a habit of doing so on a regular basis!

167

Big Sugar

This section is not so much about teaching you something that you can use to control your diet or exercise, but more of a history about nutrition. Have you ever heard the phrase "follow the money"? This phrase is often used to point towards what a particular motivation might be. In the research field sometimes you can "follow the money" to find the motivation behind the research. Sometimes the motivation can show that the results of the research might be a little skewed to favor a particular point of view or outcome. This happened in the 1960's with research around the link between heart disease and sugar.

The fight between which is worse for you fats or sugars has been going on for decades. Prior to reading this book and the sections on both fats and sugars you might have had an idea in your head about which was worse for you. Now we know that too much of either is a bad thing but the fight between the two keeps going strong in today's society. But where did this fight start? In the 1960's an organization known as the Sugar Research Foundation paid three Harvard scientists to publish a review of research done on fats and sugars relation to heart disease. That doesn't sound too bad does it? A review of research should show a variety of results that would allow you to make a rather accurate conclusion on the subject. Well that's what most people assumed, however there was a problem. The Sugar Research Foundation hand selected what research the scientists were to review, which means in the end they were able to put the blame of which is worse for your heart on dietary fats.

Now we do know that too much of either can be a bad thing and too much fatty food can have negative effects on your heart. However the problem was that when the focus was placed on fats and not sugars people replaced their food choices with low fat high sugar foods. Many experts now blame this research for the rise in obesity and obesity related problems. The Sugar Research Foundation, now known as the Sugar Association has since admitted that during the time of the research there was no requirement to reveal funding behind research and has stated they should have been more transparent about the review.

The results of the review have been the cornerstone of several nutritional guidelines and set back research on sugar decades. Although we are catching up on the issues now, the damage has already been done to millions of people. It is important to look at who is funding the research that we read, not everything is a conspiracy to fool the public into using or not using a certain product, but sometimes that is the result! For example it was shown in a New York Times article that Coca-Cola was funding the research of a group looking to downplay the link between sugary sodas and obesity. This does not mean that Coca-Cola was attempting to fool anyone. It is more likely that if the research panned out in their favor then it was worth the investment, if it didn't well then nothing really changes because people already know that soda and obesity could be linked. The point of this section is to show you that just because you removed something that was unhealthy, that doesn't mean you replaced it with something any better. Like those who replaced fats with sugar due to the research, both have their own problems and over consumption of either will lead to negative effects on your health!

168

Eating Healthy is to Expensive

Pop quiz time! How do you lose weight? Did you say eating fewer calories than you burn? Ok that was a very easy quiz, yet this section will be dedicated to a myth that tries to undermine the calories in vs calories out. The myth is that it is too expensive to eat healthy. Now this is being applied to the idea that it is too expensive to eat healthy and thus weight loss is not possible. A myth, that for whatever reason runs counter to the very concept that it is trying to promote.

The idea is that healthy food has fewer calories and that means that you are able to lose weight from eating it. Essentially the myth is admitting that in order to lose weight you have to consume fewer calories than you burn. So the myth is sort of correct. Now, think about what we have learned over the last 5 months. First does "healthy food" always have fewer calories? Is "healthy food" needed for weight loss? The answer to both of those questions is an easy no. As long as the food you eat during the day contains less calories than your body burns you will have weight loss. Admittedly you could run risk of becoming malnourished due to a lack of nutrients in junk foods, but weigh loss is still occurring all the same. With proper planning you can still select foods that are not considered "healthy" and still meet your nutritional needs and remain in your caloric deficit.

Now for the other part of the myth, that healthy food is too expensive. Research done by the Harvard School of Public Health showed that healthy food options are a little more expensive per day than the unhealthy options, totaling in at an extra $1.50 a day for the healthier options. This works out to be $550 dollars more a year for the healthier food purchases. That seems to be pointing to the idea that the myth is true, healthier food is more expansive! The study was done by reviewing 27 studies in 10 different countries. The researchers compared the cost of the unhealthiest foods and the healthiest foods to determine the cost difference. Hmm did that last statement tip you off to something? If not go back and reread it. The researchers compared the cost of the unhealthiest to the healthiest. So they took the two extremes from each group to come up with the difference of a dollar fifty a day in price.

What does this tell us about the cost difference of healthy foods and unhealthy foods? That when you come to the middle of the two groups the cost difference will be much smaller or even nonexistent! Think of when you purchased foods before you changed your diet. Did you always buy the unhealthiest foods you could find? Probably not, most of your food choices albeit unhealthy were probably in the middle of the road between the unhealthiest and the healthy selections. The same can probably be said following your switch to a new healthier diet. You probably do not purchase the healthiest most expensive food at the store. You likely are still shopping in the middle of the road, but now it is between the lower healthy foods and the healthiest ones. This means that the cost of your foods likely did not change a great deal.

Now following the idea that you might end up spending and $550 dollars a year on food for many that could be too much. For many, money can be tight and spending an extra 500 on food even over the course of a year is just too much. Consider this, research has shown that yearly medical expenses for those who are overweight average a little over $250 a year and for those who are obese the average direct medical expenses total to over $1700 a year! Looking at that an overweight person who cleans up their diet and gets to a normal weight could reduce their yearly direct medical costs by over $250 dollars a year. That could help to offset the price of the healthier food options! For those who are obese just getting your weight down to the overweight category could save you over $1000 dollars in direct medical costs, and getting your weight down to a normal level could reduce your medical costs by $1,700 dollars! That means that you could end up saving over $1,000 dollars by eating healthy and losing weight!

In the end the myth that eating healthy is more expensive is somewhat true. You can lose weight without having to switch to a healthier diet but you might find it harder to reduce calories and get the nutrients that you need. On the other hand research has shown that healthier foods could cost you and extra $1.50 a day but that was the results of comparing the two extreme ends of unhealthy and healthy. It is likely that when you compare the cost of the foods that are more middle ground of unhealthy and healthy the cost difference will be reduced or even disappears. Finally the cost of healthier food could be offset by a reduction in the average direct medical expenses of those who are overweight and obese if weight loss is achieved! Just something to consider going forward.

169

GMO

We have covered several different myths and other things about health and nutrition in this book. Some of the concepts have been based on fact others have been based on speculation or faulty research. So where do GMO's fall? It has become more and more popular for products to boast that they contain Non-GMO ingredients. Now does this mean that GMO's are bad and we should avoid them in our diets?

Let's start with defining what GMO stands for. A GMO is a Genetically Modified Organism. For most people when they think about a GMO they think that it basically only pertains to plants. However an organism is not just a plant. So a GMO could be a modified virus or bacteria and so on. Now naturally, given the subject of this book we will be focusing on the concept of GMO's in the foods that we eat. Next let's go over what actually takes place when creating a GMO. When we talk about genetics, simply we are talking about the things that make you, you. This is your DNA which contains your genes. A scientist will take the DNA from a single cell and replace a single gene in the DNA, modifying its structure and code. The vast majority of the DNA remains unchanged. Once the DNA has been changed scientist will promote the natural growth of the cell through cell division. Eventually the single cell will grow and expand to be the entire plant with the same modified DNA.

There are a few factors that farmers have to worry about when they are planting their crops; bugs weeds and weather are the main concerns effecting crop yield. This is where the majority of genetic modifications are used. Some plants might be modified to repel certain insects! This can help to reduce the use of pesticides, which both helps to reduce chemicals on our foods and overall cost of growing. Some plants might be modified so that they can grow in hotter or colder climates, or areas with limited rain fall. This allows for places with difficult conditions to grow their own foods, which could greatly help countries with fewer resources available to them.

Ok, so GMO's don't sound too bad. Do they have negative effects on our health? Well, the answer is more than likely no there are not negative effects on our health. However GMO's are new and we do not have a lot of research on the use and effects of them. So why is the answer there are no effects on our health? Think of it this way, a corn stalk contains 32,000 genes in it; when a scientist genetically modifies the corn they are changing 1 or 2 genes. This means that 32,998 – 32,999 genes remain the same as they always were. Now the genes are not modified without thorough research into what the genes being modified will do differently. This means that careful thought and precautions are taken to ensure that the genes being modified do not change things that could cause issues like allergic reactions in humans.

The National Academy for Science has concluded that GMO's are safe for human health. They have found that in the over 2 decades GMO technology has been used there have been no cases of negative effects on human health. So it is likely that when people are afraid of GMO's in their foods that they are more afraid of the idea of the foods being modified than actual cases of negative effects on humans.

170

Non-GMO

In the last section we went over what a GMO is and if they are something that you should avoid or not. In this section we will be looking at Non-GMO foods, or those that do not have any genetic modifications. This category can actually be broken down into a few categories that we will cover over this section and the following sections.

You might have noticed in the food section of the super market that there are packages that state clearly that they contain no GMO's or that they are Non-GMO. It is a way to easily identify foods that have not been modified. However it is also a marketing tool. Not containing GMO ingredients or foods has been associated with being healthier and when a product makes the statement that they are Non-GMO typically they are trying to play on the idea that if we want to be healthier we should use this product instead of the ones that contain GMO's. Although part of it is marketing there are people who are against GMO foods and prefer to purchase products that do not contain them. The last section showed that the evidence points towards GMO's are safe, but that does not mean that people are not concerned about the possible side effects. Remember GMO's have not been around for all that long and we do not know for certain the long term effects.

Basically this will come down to your personal preference. If you are ok with GMO's in your food then you will likely not be concerned about possible long term effects. If you are someone that is not sure about the use of GMO's in your food then you will likely consume Non-GMO specific products. The requirements to be Non-GMO are simple but strict. There can be no GMO's used in any stage of production. This includes the meats that you purchase. In order for a meat or poultry product to be classified as Non-GMO that animal must not consume food that contains GMO's. The plants and feed that the animals consume must also be GMO free! No stage of growth or production may have GMO's, it's that simple.

Many people will associate GMO free foods to be more natural and healthier for the body. I am not going to attempt to swing you in either direction though. Take a look at the research for yourself. Weigh the pros and the cons, and remember to look at the groups that might be funding the research or the methods they use. If the funding is bias then the results could be as well. Cross reference what you learn with a variety of sources! This will allow you to make an educated decision on where you stand with GMO and Non-GMO products. If you remain unsure consult with your doctor on what the best option is for you.

171

Organic

Organic foods are very popular in society today, but they are very popular in the health community now. To be labeled organic foods need to meet some very strict guidelines. However is organic any better for you or is it just a marketing tool? Let's take a look!

Let's begin by defining what organic actually is as it pertains to the food we eat. *"Yielding the use of food produced with the use of feed or fertilizer of plant or animal origins without employment of chemically formulated fertilizers, growth stimulants, antibiotics, or pesticides."* Basically it means that the food is grown or produced without man made products like pesticides or growth hormones. This is considered mostly an all-natural approach that is chemical free. The idea sounds great, eating food that does not contain any harmful chemicals like pesticides or other human interventions. It is also important to note that all organic foods are Non-GMO, but not all Non-GMO foods are organic! If you are concerned about the use of chemicals and antibiotics in your foods then going organic might be for you!

However, is organic better for you? From a nutritional standpoint the answer is no. When we compare the micro and macro nutrients of organic and non-organic foods they are very similar and show no real discernable difference. You will get the same nutrients from eating an organic apple as you will a non-organic one. So what about the health concerns around the chemicals and hormones/antibiotics? At this time there does not appear to be any evidence that the non-organic foods cause any health problems. Non-organic foods have been tested and have shown that their level of pesticide residue and other add ins are within safe ranges for human consumption. That being said the verdict is still out on the long term health concerns around pesticides because of the numerous environmental variables involved in food production. It is very difficult to narrow down any health related problem to prove it was caused by the pesticide or other products.

Like the GMO Non-GMO fight, it will likely come down to your personal preference! At this time organic doesn't show any benefits in nutrition over non-organic; showing that organic is not more nutritional for your body. Research has not shown that the use of pesticides or other products have caused health related concerns. But, further research is being done to look into the possibility of long term health issues. Keep in mind that if you find yourself wanting to switch to organic foods you will likely be increasing your food costs. Organic foods have been shown to cost 10-50 percent more than their non-organic counter parts! Like the last section, do your own research and make an educated decision on what you feel is best for your body! For me personally I will occasionally buy organic and Non-GMO and I will also buy non-organic and GMO products. You might find that you are ok with certain foods being non-organic while other foods you would prefer organic or Non-GMO. It is your personal preference! If you want the healthier diet that you have been working on for the last 5 months to last then it needs to be something that you enjoy and can sustain for the long term!

172

Muscles of the Body: Bicep

The Biceps is one muscle that everyone loves to work out, however this is mostly just for the glamor of them. Big biceps are often times associated with being strong or physically fit. So it is no wonder that when people go to the gym the bicep curl is one of the most popular exercises you will see being performed. Let's take a look at some of the specifics around the bicep muscle.

The bicep muscle can be found on the front of the upper arm. Its function is to flex the arm at the elbow joint as well as supinate the forearm. Supination of the forearm is when your arm is turned so your palms face up. The bicep starts in the scapula and attaches in the forearm and has what is known as 2 heads. The bicep branches out into the long head and the short head and each of these heads of the bicep are attached at different points on your scapula. The long head section is the outer section of the arm while the short head is the inner section. Because of these different points of attachments there is some debate on what is the best way to activate them in exercise.

Like any muscle in the body the bicep can be strengthened through resistance training. Some of the most well-known exercises are ones we have already covered, the standard bicep curl and the chin up. It is believed that the best way to activate the long head of the bicep is to have the elbows pulled back behind the body. The short head is thought to receive the most activation when the elbows are out in front of the body. Examples of this would be doing standard bicep curl while using a bench to place your elbows out in front of you. This is known as the preacher curls and could target the short head of the bicep more. Using a cable machine or resistance bands you can try to target the long head by standing out in front with your back to the resistance. This position will allow you to perform the exercise with your elbows behind the body. Another theory on how to activate the different heads is through the hand placement. Having a fully supinated hand during the exercise will target the short head. While having a partially supinated hand grip, or when your palms face inward towards the body, will activate the long head of the bicep.

The more you know about the muscles of your body the more efficient your workouts can become. If you are looking to develop a specific muscles or regions of the body research what is the best way to activate it. Doing your research can help to prevent injury and give you the best exercises to fully activate a muscle and force its growth, resulting in better results in less time! In some cases the phrase "work smarter not harder" can be applied.

Low Blood Sugar

In this book we have covered all sorts of problems associated with high blood sugar, now what happens when our blood sugar drops to low? There can be several causes of low blood sugar that include not consuming enough sugar, certain medications, insulin over production, other issues include hormone problems. Low blood sugar is also known by the name Hypoglycemia.

Some of the symptoms that are associated with low blood sugar levels are irregular heart rhythm, fatigue, pale skin, shakiness, sweating, frequent urination, and irritability. As the condition worsens confusion or abnormal behaviors might occur. Your vision might become blurred and you could even lose consciousness! Someone suffering from hypoglycemia might even appear to be intoxicated as they become clumsy and slur their speech. Usually the symptoms can be reversed through eating or drinking high sugar foods like candy or drinking fruit juices like orange juice.

Over time you could develop hypoglycemic unawareness which is when your body will no longer produce the signs and symptoms of low blood sugar. Although this might sound like a welcomed relief for anyone who has the symptoms regularly, it can actually be very dangerous! The symptoms are the body's way of warning you that your blood sugar is getting to low. If you no longer display the symptoms then you are at risk of life threatening conditions. If you are someone who believes they are experiencing the symptoms of hypoglycemia please contact your doctor immediately! Some ways that you can prevent hypoglycemia is to eat small frequent meals throughout the day. This prevents the body's blood sugar from dropping to much between meals. Keep in mind that this is not a good long term strategy; discuss the issue with your doctor to address the underlying causes of hypoglycemia.

Exercises Effects on Cognitive Function

I have harped on the benefits of being physically active and exercising over the last (almost) 6 months. In all that time the benefits of regular exercise have been explained to only show the physical benefits. Benefits like stronger heart, stronger muscle, increased flexibility and joint mobility to name a few. However there is another benefit that we have not covered yet; that is the effects regular exercise has on your cognitive function!

The research is very clear on this, exercise helps with brain function. But How? One study by the University of British Columbia showed that regular aerobic exercise increased the size of the hippocampus in the brain. This is the area of the brain that is responsible for verbal memory and our ability to learn. It has also been shown that exercising following learning helps to boost retention of the new information. For someone in the Health and PE field, this fact is our biggest argument for daily physical education for all students. Taking a little time out of the school day to promote moderate exercise could help students to retain what they are taught in their core classes as well as set them up with lifelong health practices.

The cognitive benefits of physical activity do not stop at just learning and memory retention! There is evidence that it can help reduce your risk of developing dementia later in life. Researchers have found that those who engaged in just leisure time physical activity at least two times a week were less likely to develop dementia in their later years. This does not mean that if you are already in "middle age" that it is too late to get the benefits of physical activity. Even waiting until midlife to begin being more physically active showed a reduction in dementia risks! This is especially true for those who are overweight or obese in their middle age.

As this book is coming to an end this was my final attempt to show the benefits of being physically active. We have gone over so many different ways to be active, by now I hope that you were able to find one that works for you! Some of you might find that you are happy lifting weights or taking brisk walks around the park. Others of you have found that outdoor activities like hiking, kayaking, or orienteering were perfect for you. If you have not found a physical activity or group of activities that you enjoy I encourage you to keep looking. Exercise is not a one size fits all thing. Some people might love the workouts that I do while others would leave the session without so much as a good bye. If you pick something that you find fun and engaging then it won't be exercise to you it will be your hobby. By this point you know the benefits of being active; you know the improvements even just 20 minutes a day can make on your life. You know that even if you are busy you need to make time in your life for your physical activity. You know you should be doing it. If you haven't yet, what are you waiting for?

175

Calorie Review

As yesterday's section was a final attempt to display the benefits of physical exercise I thought I would take today to review some of the content that we covered earlier in this book. It will be a nice short section, but hopefully it will just refresh your memory and help to set you up for long term success after you close this book for the last time in a week.

All calories are equal when it comes to energy. This is something that we have gone over several times throughout these pages. Your body does not care if it is storing excess calories from celery or from ice cream. If you eat more calories than you burn they will get stored as fat cells all the same. Often times you will find articles and opinions stating that not all calories are equal; but it is important to look into what they are claiming is not equal between calories. The all calories are not equal is correct in one sense but not in all. When we are talking about a calorie by its most basic definition they are all the same because a calorie is just a unit of measurement of energy. An example I gave to you at the start of this book was that your TV doesn't care how your energy is created because a unit of energy to it is the same whether it came from a wind turbine or a coal plant. A joule is a joule a watt is a watt. However there is a way that the all calories are not equal statement is true!

Remember a calorie is made up of all of carbohydrates, proteins, and fats in the food you eat. Not all calories contain the same amount of each of these 3 ingredients and therefore the nutrition gained from a calorie can be different. Some calories could be 85% carbohydrates, 5% protein and 5% fat. While another could be 50% protein and 50% fat. These nutrients have different functions in our bodies and we have a need in our bodies to have a certain percentage of them to make up part of our daily diet. As I briefly mention before, digestion consumes a certain amount of energy in the body, some estimates show that a person uses about 10% of their daily energy on the digestive process alone. During digestion however, each of the three nutrients that make up a calorie cost a different amount of energy to digest. Protein takes the most energy, burning about 20-30% of what you ate to digest while carbohydrates take between 5-10% to digest. Fats take the least amount of energy at up to 3% burned during digestion. In the end a diet higher in protein means that you are not absorbing as much energy because your body has to work harder to break it down and digest it. Think of this like taxes in your paycheck, you earned all of the money but some of it is taken out in taxes. When you eat you get all of the calories but some of them are used to break down and digest what you ate.

A calorie is a calorie is a calorie, when it comes to energy. However when it comes to nutrition not all calories are the same, and some are better for you than others. This is why it is so important to focus on eating healthy during weight loss. Yes you can lose weight no matter what you eat as long as you eat fewer calories than you need but you might not get the nourishment that you need! Keep an eye on what you eat and you will lose weight, have more energy and just all around feel better because your body is getting what it needs to thrive!

176

Rest Time Between Exercises

One of the things that people often get wrong when they are at the gym or doing their own exercise routine is how much rest time do you take between exercises. For many people they either take too long of a rest period or not long enough. But what is the ideal rest time?

In reality this is a question that has multiple answers because it can be asked in multiple ways. We are going to briefly cover a few ways this question can be asked and what the answers could be. The first way to ask the question is how much time you should take between exercise sessions for a muscle group. This is a pretty easy answer and I have mentioned it in prior sections. It is recommended that you take 24 to 48 hours to rest the muscles that you worked out before exercising them again. Why though? When the muscle is worked out through resistance microscopic tears can occur in the muscle tissue as well as damage to the contractile portion of the muscles known as the myosin head and actin filament. When a muscle contracts it is actually tiny "hooks" called myosin that attach to the actin and walk or row the muscle fibers causing the contraction. It takes time for your body to repair these tears and fix the myosin/actin systems.

Another way this question can be asked is how long to take between sets of the same exercise. This version of the question is just as important as the other version. Some people will say you need to take 30 seconds between sets while others say you should be taking 5 minutes. You will notice in the gym that people don't really time their rest but more go by a feeling. "I feel ready to do another set". Using a feeling is typically a good way to measure your rest time but it can cause you to take too much time between sets. Taking too much time between sets can reduce the benefits of the exercise. Remember resistance training like weight lifting relies on the anaerobic system for energy. Too much rest between sets will reduce the potential for improving your anaerobic endurance. On the other end not taking enough time between sets would prevent you from rebuilding your energy stores and result in reduced performance. For most people and beginners you should aim for 45 seconds to 2 minutes of rest between sets.

The last version of the question that I am going to cover is; how long to rest between doing one exercise and then a different exercise? The answer to this really depends on what exercise you completed and what one you are moving onto. If you are going from one exercise to another that works out the same muscle or muscle group then you should still follow the 45 seconds to 2 minutes guidelines. If you are moving to an exercise that works out a different muscle than the previous exercise then you could move right into it without much rest. When people perform circuit training they will typically have each exercise workout a different muscle so that they can move right from one exercise to another without rest because the next muscle should not be fatigued and be ready to go.

Each person is different however; your ideal rest time can change. If the exercise you are doing is explosive and requires a lot of energy, such as deadlifting, then you might need some more rest time between sets or exercises. If the exercise you are doing is light then you might want to aim for the lower end of the guidelines. Do what works for you but keep the guidelines in mind, they could help you to achieve the best results for the time you put in. You want to be efficient with a workout, and your rest time is part of that. Let's put it into an example. We covered the fitness program "Strong Lifts 5x5", and in this program you perform 3 exercises for 5 sets of 5 repetitions each. For the sake of the example and easy math let's assume that the actual exercise takes 1 minute per set. For the workout there are a total of 15 sets, so 15 total minutes of exercising. If you were to take a minute of rest between each set then that is an additional 15 minutes of rest time brining your workout time to 30 minutes. Now take the same workout and make the rest time 3 minutes long. Your total rest time would be 45 minutes and your exercise time would remain 15 minutes. The difference is now your workout is an hour long instead of 30 minutes! Rest time is as important for your muscles as it is for your schedule!

Calorie Tip: Plate Size

There is something about human nature that when you have a plate you fill the whole plate with food. So it would stand to reason that if you have a larger plate then you will fill it with more food. Using a smaller plate might help you to maintain portion control because you are not able to put as much food on it.

Research done by Cornell University found that reducing the size of the plate from a 12 inch dinner plate to a 10 inch plate resulted in a reduction in calories consumed by 22%. I want you to think on that for a moment. If your dinner was 800 calories then reducing the calorie count by 22% means that the dinner would now be 624 calories. That is a reduction of 176 calories for a single large meal! Remember what I said about how much weight you would gain per year by over eating by only 100 calories a day? It is believed that the reducing plate size results in eating less because of something known as the Delboeuf Illusion. This is the idea that things appear smaller when compared to something bigger. Basically you think that your portion is smaller when on a larger plate so you end up increasing portion size. On the other side if your plate is smaller than your portion sizes will appear larger even if they are not.

It might seem so simple that you might think that it couldn't possible affect you but in reality there is a reason why things like the Delboeuf Illusion exist. Things could affect you without you ever even knowing it! If you are finding that you are struggling with portion size or you are beginning to trust yourself to "eyeball" your portion sizes, using smaller plates could help you to keep your portion sizes down. Making small changes to different areas in your life can result in some big improvements!

Taking a Break

If you have been following along faithfully then you will be coming up on 6 months of hard work. You have been changing your diet and maintaining that change. You have been working on improving your fitness and working out. 178 days of continuous hard work is an amazing thing to accomplish. Some of you might have achieved your goal already while some of you will still have some work to do. One of the problems is how much longer is it going to take?

I have referred to this process as a marathon and not a sprint several times over the course of this book. For some of you that marathon might be very long, it all depends on what your starting weight is compared to your goal weight. 6 months is a long time but it might not be long enough for you to reach your goal. Sometimes it might be necessary for you to take a short break and get yourself back in the right mindset to keep going.

Now when I say take a break I do not mean that you should go back to your old habits! Going back to your old habits will do nothing but undo some of the progress that you made. Being in a constant calorie deficit can be very difficult and maintaining one for a long period of time can be even harder. If you take a break from your calorie deficit it is important not to go into a calorie surplus! Reassess your TDEE and find out how many calories you need to maintain at your current weight. This will tell you how many calories you can eat on average per day to maintain whatever weight you are at. This is known as the maintenance phase, and you will be in this phase for the rest of your life once you reach your goal. The maintenance phase is when you find a balance by consuming the amount of calories your body needs to perform its day to day functions but not so many that you accumulate fat storages.

If you find yourself needing a break then enter your maintenance phase so that your weight loss will stop or slow down but you will not gain the weight that you lost back. When in the maintenance phase you are able to eat a little more food because you are no longer running on a calorie deficit. However I do not recommend that you remain on this break for long if you are still trying to reach your goal weight. Although you will not be gaining your weight back you will not be losing any either. Staying in the maintenance phase for too long before you reach your goal weight will not only push back the date you wanted to reach your goal but it could also make it more difficult to get yourself back on your calorie deficit to continue to lose weight. Short breaks might help to get you motivated and feel "recharged", but taking short breaks to often will also mean it will take longer for you to reach your goal. It is a balance that you need to find. You might never feel like you need a break or you might feel like you need one once or twice a year. Either way if you take a break be smart about it! Don't return to old habits and don't hurt the progress you already made!

179

Make your Maintenance Phase Easier

Ok, so I may or may not have lied to you a few sections back when I said that I was done trying to push the importance of physical activity on you. Towards the end of writing this it was hard to decide exactly what I wanted to include or exclude in the final pages. The last section mentioning maintenance phase made me want to add in one last thing about physical activity.

As you have learned the maintenance phase is when you balance your calories in vs calories out. You will not gain or lose any weight in this phase, although your weight might fluctuate a little it will remain the same on average. One of the best ways to help you in your maintenance phase is to exercise a little every day. I have stated the health benefits of exercise as often as I have stated the benefits of a healthy diet. However this section has nothing to do with the health benefits of exercise; it is all about the calories burnt! All movements require calories to be burnt and exercise typically involves a lot of movement. Some exercises can burn a lot of calories in a short amount of time while others take a little longer to reach the same number of calories. For example, hitting the heavy bag for a half hour a day could burn anywhere from 150 to 300 calories for an average size person. Walking for the same amount of time might burn 100 to 150 calories depending on your size and pace.

Burning extra calories during the maintenance phase through exercise is a way for you to increase the amount of food that you are able to eat! Think about it for a moment, if you burnt an extra 250 calories a day through exercise that could allow you to increase the amount of food you can consume during the day or else you will lose weight because you would be back in a calorie deficit if you don't consume the calories you burnt! Remember back to all the times you have assessed your TDEE; you had to select an activity level to plug into your math equation. The more active you are the more calories you burnt throughout the day! Increasing your activity increases you TDEE which in turn means that you can eat a little more throughout the day without gaining weight!

180

Red Meat

I have covered all sorts of different diets and foods that have an impact on your health so far, you might have been surprised that I didn't cover red meat earlier. We have all heard about how diets high in red meats or processed meats increase your risk of heart disease and maybe even cancer, so why didn't I cover it sooner? Don't worry this isn't a trick question; I am not going to tell you that the research shows it is perfectly healthy for you. But I am going to cover it in a little better light than what some of the research would have you believe.

Some of the research has shown that those who eat more red or processed meats might be increasing their risk of death by 13 to 20 percent. One study followed 121,000 people for an average of 24 years, and every 4 years the subjects would submit information about their diets. During the time of the study almost 24,000 of the participants died. The results showed that those who ate more meats died at a higher rate. That seems pretty conclusive doesn't it?

Take what you have already learned throughout this book and apply it to the study that I mentioned. What have you picked up on? First the diets were self-reported and we know that people are very bad at reporting their diets so some of the information could be a little skewed. That doesn't mean that the findings were wrong though. Secondly what do we know about red meats and processed meats? They can be high in saturated fats, cholesterol and sodium. So it is likely that the causes of any health issues when it comes to the red meats are found in the levels of saturated fats and sodium. Meats contain these nutrients so it is safe to say that over eating red or processed meats will cause you to surpass your daily recommended amounts!

If you enjoy eating red meats then you will likely be ok to keep doing so as long as you are staying within the recommended daily amount for the nutrients that the meats contain. I should also note that other long term studies have shown no link to moderate daily meat consumption (3 ounces of meat a day) and premature death. This tells me that it is likely that red meat could be part of a nutritional problem but not the only culprit. Maintaining a balanced diet, even one that includes red meats will ensure that your body is getting the correct nutrients that it needs. Over consumption of certain nutrients, like those found in red meats, could lead to health issues! This seems to be another case that supports eating in moderation and not following restrictive dieting.

181

Gluten Free

Although the gluten free craze seems to be coming to an end, it is still something out there that people believe will make them healthier. You are on day 181 so I am sure that by now you might have figured out that the gluten free diet really was no different from the other restrictive diets you see out there. However could going gluten free if you do not suffer from celiac disease harm you?

Celiac disease is a condition where people who eat gluten will trigger the body to attack the small intestines. This attack by their own body can cause inflammation, malnutrition, and gastrointestinal distress. Although gluten has been made out to be some big bad guy in every ones diets all it really is, is a protein found in wheat and barley. For people who have celiac disease cutting out gluten will stop the body from attacking the small intestines and prevent the resulting symptoms. It is likely that gluten has gotten a bad name because the body's attacks on the small intestines can actually increase the risk of heart disease for those with celiac. Do those who do not have the condition still need to worry about the increased risk of heart disease?

The answer seems to be a no. A study that followed 110,000 people for 25 years found that there was no difference in rate of heart attack between those who ate the most gluten and those who ate the least amount of gluten. However the results did show that those who avoided gluten by cutting out whole grains had an increased risk of heart disease. Why might this be? Well as you have learned the whole grains can be what we call nutrient dense, meaning they contain valuable nutrients. Cutting out these nutrients is not good for your heart health, so in the end if you do not have celiac disease then cutting out gluten could actually be bad for you!

Much like almost all fad diet trends there is little evidence to back them up. Unless you have celiac disease gluten will not harm you and you will not receive any extra health benefits by cutting it out. The only people that actually benefitted from the anti-gluten diet trend were those with celiac disease. Although I am sure it was very annoying for them to watch people go gluten free for the wrong reasons, they did have the added benefit of raised awareness. Restaurants increased their gluten free menus and grocery stores added in gluten free aisles, giving them more food options. However in the end gluten is not bad and you really do not need to avoid it unless you have celiac. If you believe you could have the condition you should consult with your doctor.

182

The End

Can you believe that you have finally reached the end of this book? If you followed along the way it was intended then 6 months have passed. When you first started reading this finishing it might have seen like a big challenge and losing weight might have seemed like an even bigger challenge! If you have followed through and applied what you have learned to fit your life then you will have accomplished two things. First you will have lost weight, improving your overall health. Second, you will have learned how to apply changes to your life that will allow you to keep the weight off for life!

Your journey does not end once you finish this section. You might be at goal weight now or you might be there in another 6 months either way what you have learned will be with you for life. Remember the goal of this book was not to prescribe you a specific diet or workout to complete but to teach you the principles of weight loss and nutrition as well as the benefits of physical activity. Applying the principles of weight loss to your individual needs and life allows you to set habits and make a life style change. When you apply what you have learned to your life it will be something that you can keep up for years to come. Unlike restrictive dieting that will always come to an end a lifestyle change will always be with you!

Once you reach your goal weight reassess your TDEE and find how many calories you need for your maintenance phase. You will strive to achieve this daily so that you will remain at your goal weight for life. Like everything else as you stay in maintenance phase for a period of time you will become use to the amount of food you can eat and will no longer need to be as strict with your calorie counting. However it is very important that you do not return to your old habits! Think about how diets fail and within 5 years most people gain the weight back, and why. If you return to old habits over a few years you could gain all of the weight right back! Those old habits made you overweight once and they will do it again!

Think of it like a bucket under a dripping faucet. The drip might not seem like a lot at first but given enough time the bucket will fill up and overflow! This is the same as your body. The dripping is you over eating by just a little and as you slowly over eat your body will fill up with fat again, like water in the bucket. In both situations it is best to just fix the problem instead of having to empty the bucket from time to time or having to lose the weight again. Fix the sink and stop over eating. Monitor your weight from time to time, try monthly, and if you notice that you have gained some of the weight back address the problem while it is only a few extra pounds. Before you know it those few extra pounds could be a few extra 10's of pounds! Like the dripping faucet, if you empty the bucket when there are only a few drops, it will be easier than waiting until it is full again.

I really hope that you found success with what you have learned from this book. Not everything will apply to you and I am sure there were sections that were redundant or you didn't enjoy, however I hope that you were able to pick up enough information to make a positive change in your life! As I said months ago, weight loss is one of the easiest things you can do, on paper. In practice it is difficult and tiresome, but by knowing how the body uses calories and nutrients will allow you to set yourself up for long term success! Although this is the end of this part of your journey you are capable of doing this on your own. Continue to monitor your calorie and nutrient intake, and keep watching your portion sizes. You will find long term success.

I will leave you with a final congratulation! What you have done in the last 6 months is no small accomplishment! Think back on where you were when you first opened this book. Were you heavier? Were you unhealthy? Were you inactive? Did you do what you could to avoid movements? Now look at where you are! Have you lost a large amount of weight? Are you stronger and fit? Do you feel healthier? Do you engage in physical activity either through planned exercise or just a more active lifestyle? You have made small changes to your life over the period of 6 months and it is likely that those small changes added up to some monumental lifestyle improvements!

Now it is on you to keep those changes going to meet your goal or to maintain at your goal. In all honesty it has been on you the whole time, I might have taught you a little or a lot along the way but it was up to you to make the changes and apply it to your life. How successful you have been or will be is all dependent on you! You have come this far and accomplished so much, so I know that you can remain successful in your new lifestyle.

So this is Goodbye for now, I hope that I was successful in helping you to help yourself.

Bibliography

"BRO SPLIT" ROUTINES: ARE THEY EFFECTIVE FOR BUILDING MUSCLE? (n.d.). Retrieved from http://seannal.com/articles/training/bro-split.php

 Retrieved from https://study.com/academy/lesson/what-is-the-latissimus-dorsi-definition-function.html

10 easy ways to work out while you work. (2017, May 10). Retrieved from https://www.mayoclinic.org/healthy-lifestyle/adult-health/in-depth/office-exercise/art-20047394

10 ways to be an expert at spotting nutrition quackery. (2015, September 02). Retrieved from https://eatwell2bewellrd.com/10-ways-to-be-an-expert-at-spotting-nutrition-quackery/

2014, 2. J. (n.d.). Salt vs. sodium: Are they the same? Retrieved from https://sodiumbreakup.heart.org/salt-vs-sodium

Ab Wheel Effectiveness - How Effective is the Ab Wheel? (2018, January 09). Retrieved from https://www.darkironfitness.com/ab-wheel-effectiveness-how-effective-ab-wheel/

ADF - Drug Facts - Caffeine. (n.d.). Retrieved from https://adf.org.au/drug-facts/caffeine/

Adipose tissue. (2018, December 10). Retrieved from https://en.wikipedia.org/wiki/Adipose_tissue

Alli weight-loss pill: How does it work and are there risks? (2018, February 06). Retrieved from https://www.mayoclinic.org/healthy-lifestyle/weight-loss/in-depth/alli/art-20047908

Anaerobic Exercise: What You Should Know. (n.d.). Retrieved from https://www.healthline.com/health/fitness-exercise/anaerobic-exercise

Anon, (2015). Fitness Components. [online] Available at: https://static.k12.com/eli/bb/1054/2_59518/1_107640_1_59519/81029a9f3d9ff9db23bc0a8b459c2e2534e86bc0/page_1.html [Accessed 25 Sep. 2018].

Antioxidants: Beyond the Hype. (2018, February 26). Retrieved from https://www.hsph.harvard.edu/nutritionsource/antioxidants/

Atkins. (n.d.). What's the Difference between Carbohydrates & Sugar on Food Labels? Retrieved from https://sa.atkins.com/blog/what's-the-difference-between-carbohydrates-and-sugar-on-food-labels/

Aubrey, A. (2013, June 26). Can You Be Addicted To Carbs? Scientists Are Checking That Out. Retrieved from https://www.npr.org/sections/thesalt/2013/06/26/195292850/can-you-be-addicted-to-carbs-scientists-are-checking-that-out

Balance Board Benefits. (n.d.). Retrieved from https://www.livestrong.com/article/34421-balance-board-benefits/

Barclay, E. (2014, June 09). Fruit Juice Vs. Soda? Both Beverages Pack In Sugar, Health Risks. Retrieved from https://www.npr.org/sections/thesalt/2014/06/09/319230765/fruit-juice-vs-soda-both-beverages-pack-in-sugar-and-health-risk

Basal metabolic rate. (2018, November 25). Retrieved from https://en.wikipedia.org/wiki/Basal_metabolic_rate

Biceps. (2018, November 27). Retrieved from https://en.wikipedia.org/wiki/Biceps

Body Fat Spot Reduction Works? Liberating Fat W/ Weight, Burning it With Cardio Training is the Key, Study Claims. (n.d.). Retrieved from http://suppversity.blogspot.com/2017/05/body-fat-spot-reduction-works.html

Bookishclaire, & KerryOK5. (2018, December 18). The Original Ranch® | Hidden Valley® Ranch. Retrieved from https://www.hiddenvalley.com/products/bottled-dressings/original-ranch/original-ranch/

Bradley, B. (2015, July 24). Are Wraps Really Healthier Than Sandwiches? Retrieved from https://www.gq.com/story/sandwiches-vs-wraps-diet-tips

Brandt, M. L. (2004, July 21). Obese parents increase kids' risk of being overweight. Retrieved from https://news.stanford.edu/news/2004/july21/med-obesity-721.html

Brazier, Y. (2017, April 26). Weight Watchers: Community, points, benefits, and planning. Retrieved from https://www.medicalnewstoday.com/articles/149454.php

Buchholz, C, A., Schoeller, & A, D. (2004, May 01). Is a calorie a calorie? Retrieved from https://academic.oup.com/ajcn/article/79/5/899S/4690223

Cadman, B. (n.d.). Visceral fat: What it is, why it is dangerous, and how to get rid of it. Retrieved from https://www.medicalnewstoday.com/articles/320929.php

Calculate TDEE – Daily Calorie Requirements. (2014, August 21). Retrieved from http://www.superskinnyme.com/calculate-tdee.html

CBSNewYork. (2011, October 25). 1 Soda A Day Equals 50 Pounds Of Sugar A Year, Says NYC Health Department. Retrieved from https://newyork.cbslocal.com/2011/10/25/1-soda-a-day-equals-50-pounds-of-sugar-a-year-says-nyc-health-department/

Center for Food Safety and Applied Nutrition. (n.d.). Labeling & Nutrition - How to Understand and Use the Nutrition Facts Label. Retrieved from https://www.fda.gov/food/labelingnutrition/ucm274593.htm#seeb

Chodosh, S. (2018, January 12). Here's why your body stores more fat in certain places. Retrieved from https://www.popsci.com/why-fat-goes-to-my-whatever#page-2

Cholesterol. (2018, October 23). Retrieved from https://medlineplus.gov/cholesterol.html

Choose your carbs wisely. (2017, February 07). Retrieved from https://www.mayoclinic.org/healthy-lifestyle/nutrition-and-healthy-eating/in-depth/carbohydrates/art-20045705

Coleman, E., & L.D. (2018, December 14). Each Gram of Protein & Carbohydrates Contains How Many Kilocalories? Retrieved from https://healthyeating.sfgate.com/gram-protein-carbohydrates-contains-many-kilocalories-5978.html

Conducting Research: The Process. (n.d.). Retrieved from https://libguides.wustl.edu/research

Core (anatomy). (2018, February 13). Retrieved from https://en.wikipedia.org/wiki/Core_(anatomy)

Crab mentality. (2018, October 22). Retrieved from https://en.wikipedia.org/wiki/Crab_mentality

Diuretics. (2016, June 10). Retrieved from https://www.mayoclinic.org/diseases-conditions/high-blood-pressure/in-depth/diuretics/art-20048129

Does Sleep Affect Weight Loss? How It Works. (n.d.). Retrieved from https://www.webmd.com/diet/sleep-and-weight-loss#1

Donnelly, L. (2016, July 28). Working in the office is as bad as smoking, study finds. Retrieved from https://www.smh.com.au/business/workplace/working-in-the-office-is-as-bad-as-smoking-study-finds-20160728-gqfcjz.html

Eating healthy vs. unhealthy diet costs about $1.50 more per day. (2014, January 13). Retrieved from https://www.hsph.harvard.edu/news/press-releases/healthy-vs-unhealthy-diet-costs-1-50-more/

Editor. (2017, September 25). Upper Back Muscles. Retrieved from http://www.medicalartlibrary.com/back-muscles/

Editors, S. (2015, December 17). Stop Hating the Scale. Retrieved from https://www.shape.com/lifestyle/mind-and-body/when-your-weight-fluctuates-whats-normal-and-whats-not

Fiber. (2018, June 06). Retrieved from https://www.hsph.harvard.edu/nutritionsource/carbohydrates/fiber/

Fitzmaurice, R. (2018, February 22). A personal trainer says taking BCAAs, supplements popular with fitness influencers, is a waste of time - here's the simple thing you should do instead. Retrieved from https://www.businessinsider.com/do-bcaa-supplements-help-performance-2018-2

Frey, M., & Fogoros, R. N. (n.d.). The Number of Calories in Popular Beers. Retrieved from https://www.verywellfit.com/diet-friendly-beer-choices-3495641

From Couch to 5K: 5 Crucial Things to Know Before You Start Training. (2018, September 28). Retrieved from https://www.nerdfitness.com/blog/couch-to-5k-crucial-things-to-know-before-you-start-training/

Fruit Juices Calories. (n.d.). Retrieved from http://www.calories.info/food/fruit-juices

Fspirvine.com. (2018). 10 Easy Ways to Increase Your NEAT (Non-exercise activity thermogenesis). [online] Available at: http://www.fspirvine.com/10-easy-ways-to-increase-your-neat/ [Accessed 25 Sep. 2018].

Greener Selection. (n.d.). Retrieved from http://www.dole.com/en/products/greener-selection

Harvard Health Publishing. (n.d.). Exercising in water: Big heart benefits and little downside. Retrieved from https://www.health.harvard.edu/exercise-and-fitness/exercising-in-water-big-heart-benefits-and-little-downside

Harvard Health Publishing. (n.d.). Get smart about treadmills. Retrieved from
https://www.health.harvard.edu/staying-healthy/get-smart-about-treadmills

Harvard Health Publishing. (n.d.). Glossary of exercise terms. Retrieved from
https://www.health.harvard.edu/newsletter_article/Glossary-of-exercise-terms

Harvard Health Publishing. (n.d.). HIT workouts may boost exercise motivation. Retrieved from
https://www.health.harvard.edu/exercise-and-fitness/hit-workouts-may-boost-exercise-motivation

Harvard Health Publishing. (n.d.). Listing of vitamins. Retrieved from
https://www.health.harvard.edu/staying-healthy/listing_of_vitamins

Harvard Health Publishing. (n.d.). New concerns about diet sodas. Retrieved from
https://www.health.harvard.edu/staying-healthy/new-concerns-about-diet-sodas

Harvard Health Publishing. (n.d.). Precious metals and other important minerals for health. Retrieved
from https://www.health.harvard.edu/staying-healthy/precious-metals-and-other-important-
minerals-for-health

Harvard Health Publishing. (n.d.). Should you go organic? Retrieved from
https://www.health.harvard.edu/staying-healthy/should-you-go-organic

Harvard Health Publishing. (n.d.). Should you take probiotics? Retrieved from
https://www.health.harvard.edu/staying-healthy/should-you-take-probiotics

Harvard Health Publishing. (n.d.). The dubious practice of detox. Retrieved from
https://www.health.harvard.edu/staying-healthy/the-dubious-practice-of-detox

Harvard Health Publishing. (n.d.). The top 5 benefits of cycling. Retrieved from
https://www.health.harvard.edu/staying-healthy/the-top-5-benefits-of-cycling

Harvard Health Publishing. (n.d.). Weight-loss surgery is an option for many. Retrieved from
https://www.health.harvard.edu/newsletter_article/Weight-loss_surgery_is_an_option_for_many

Harvard Health Publishing. (n.d.). What's the beef with red meat? Retrieved from
https://www.health.harvard.edu/healthbeat/whats-the-beef-with-red-meat

Harvard Health Publishing. (n.d.). Yoga – Benefits Beyond the Mat. Retrieved from
https://www.health.harvard.edu/staying-healthy/yoga-benefits-beyond-the-mat

Helmer, J. (n.d.). Zumba: Benefits and What to Expect. Retrieved from
https://www.webmd.com/fitness-exercise/a-z/zumba-workouts

Here's What Sitting for Long Periods of Time Does to Your Body. (n.d.). Retrieved from
https://fitness.mercola.com/sites/fitness/archive/2015/05/08/sitting-too-long.aspx

High blood pressure (hypertension). (2018, May 12). Retrieved from
https://www.mayoclinic.org/diseases-conditions/high-blood-pressure/symptoms-causes/syc-
20373410

How Long Does it Take for Something to Become a Habit? (n.d.). Retrieved from
https://examinedexistence.com/how-long-does-it-take-for-something-to-become-a-habit/

How Many Calories Does Digestion Use Up? (n.d.). Retrieved from
https://www.livestrong.com/article/320370-how-many-calories-does-digestion-use-up/

Hr.virginia.edu. (2018). [online] Available at:
http://www.hr.virginia.edu/uploads/documents/media/Writing_SMART_Goals.pdf [Accessed 25
Sep. 2018].

Hughes, L. (n.d.). How Many Calories Are in Your Wine? Retrieved from
https://www.webmd.com/diet/features/how-many-calories-in-wine

Human nutrition. (2018, December 02). Retrieved from
https://en.wikipedia.org/wiki/Human_nutrition

Hypertension and Obesity: How Weight-loss Affects Hypertension. (n.d.). Retrieved from
https://www.obesityaction.org/community/article-library/hypertension-and-obesity-how-weight-
loss-affects-hypertension/

Hypoglycemia. (2018, September 07). Retrieved from https://www.mayoclinic.org/diseases-
conditions/hypoglycemia/symptoms-causes/syc-20373685

InBody USA. (2018). What Walking 10,000 Steps Does (and doesn't) Do For You - InBody USA.
[online] Available at: https://inbodyusa.com/blogs/inbodyblog/99465793-what-walking-10-000-
steps-does-and-doesn-t-do-for-you/ [Accessed 25 Sep. 2018].

Is sweating a sign of a good workout? (2017, May 08). Retrieved from
https://www.health24.com/Lifestyle/Healthy-you/is-sweating-a-sign-of-a-good-workout-20170508

Isolated on white nutrition facts label. Eps8. (n.d.). Retrieved from
https://www.istockphoto.com/vector/nutrition-facts-label-isolated-on-white-gm470869444-
63199077

James Clear. (2018, August 07). Feeling Fat? Use These 2 Easy Ways to Lose Weight. Retrieved from
https://jamesclear.com/feeling-fat

Kim, J. (2017, March 13). PPL Routines: A Definitive Guide To Push, Pull, and Legs Splits. Retrieved
from http://hackyour.fitness/ppl-routines-definitive-guide-push-pull-legs-splits/

Knapton, S. (2018, November 25). Children mirror weight gain and losses of their mothers but not
fathers. Retrieved from https://www.telegraph.co.uk/science/2018/11/25/d/

L.D., K. Z. (2018, April 13). Can protein shakes help with weight loss? Retrieved from
https://www.mayoclinic.org/healthy-lifestyle/weight-loss/expert-answers/protein-shakes/faq-
20058335

LD, M. W. (2017, June 20). Kiwifruit: Health benefits and nutritional information. Retrieved from
https://www.medicalnewstoday.com/articles/271232.php

Levine, J. (2002). Non-exercise activity thermogenesis (NEAT). Best Practice & Research Clinical Endocrinology & Metabolism, 16(4), pp.679-702.

Luff, C. (2018). How Can You Easily Calculate Your Target Heart Rate?. [online] Verywell Fit. Available at: https://www.verywellfit.com/how-to-calculate-your-target-heart-rate-zone-2911283 [Accessed 25 Sep. 2018].

Lynch, K., Sutton, R., Michigan State University Extension, & CMU. (2018, October 02). Everything you need to know about fiber. Retrieved from http://www.canr.msu.edu/news/everything_you_need_to_know_about_fiber

Matthews, M. (2018, September 06). Does Electrical Muscle Stimulation Work? What the Science Actually Says. Retrieved from https://www.muscleforlife.com/does-electrical-muscle-stimulation-work-what-the-science-actually-says/

McDonald's Nutrition Calculator | McDonald's. (n.d.). Retrieved from https://www.mcdonalds.com/us/en-us/about-our-food/nutrition-calculator.html

Mehdi. (2018, December 21). StrongLifts 5×5: Get Stronger by Lifting Weights only 3x/Week. Retrieved from https://stronglifts.com/5x5/#gref

Muscle Memory: Why It's Easier to Get Into Shape the Second Time Around. (2011, December 04). Retrieved from https://cathe.com/muscle-memory-why-its-easier-to-get-into-shape-the-second-time-around/

Natural and Added Sugars: Two Sides of the Same Coin. (2015, October 05). Retrieved from http://sitn.hms.harvard.edu/flash/2015/natural-and-added-sugars-two-sides-of-the-same-coin/

Nippard, J. (2018, July 30). Why You Don't Need 8 Glasses of Water a Day (Does Coffee Count?). Retrieved from https://www.youtube.com/watch?v=d9dq-yQVqCU&list=PLp4G6oBUcv8w7mOuaiouhArVD2J4JMW5Z&index=21

Nippard, J. (2018, June 26). How To Lose Bodyfat From Specific Bodyparts (Why It's Possible). Retrieved from https://www.youtube.com/watch?v=XM1JPtF_vdA&index=19&list=PLp4G6oBUcv8w7mOuaiouhArVD2J4JMW5Z

Nippard, J. (2018). IS "STARVATION MODE" A REAL THING? (What The Science Says). [video] Available at: https://www.youtube.com/watch?v=1a8zuTfZhK0 [Accessed 25 Sep. 2018].

Nordqvist, C. (2017, July 17). 9 most popular diets rated by experts 2017. Retrieved from https://www.medicalnewstoday.com/articles/5847.php

Nordqvist, C. (2017, March 10). Vegetarian diet: Benefits, risks, and tips. Retrieved from https://www.medicalnewstoday.com/articles/8749.php

Parker-Pope, T. (2011, May 25). Less Active at Work, Americans Have Packed on Pounds. Retrieved from https://well.blogs.nytimes.com/2011/05/25/less-active-at-work-americans-have-packed-on-pounds/

Parker, S. (2013). The human body book. New York: DK, pp.120-121, 134-135.

Pedersen, D. (2007, June 25). Portion Control Plate for Weight Loss in Obese Patients With Type 2 Diabetes Mellitus. Retrieved from https://jamanetwork.com/journals/jamainternalmedicine/fullarticle/412650

Perry, M. (2018). How To Do A Push-Up With Proper Form (& Technique). [online] BuiltLean. Available at: https://www.builtlean.com/2011/02/23/how-to-proper-push-up-form/ [Accessed 25 Sep. 2018].

Physical Activity Improves Cognitive Function. (n.d.). Retrieved from https://www.psychologytoday.com/us/blog/the-athletes-way/201404/physical-activity-improves-cognitive-function

Portion control guide. (n.d.). Retrieved from http://diet.mayoclinic.org/diet/eat/portion-control-guide?xid=nl_MayoClinicDiet_20141027

Praderio, C. (2016, October 10). I spent a week using an under-the-desk cycle - here's what it was like. Retrieved from https://www.businessinsider.com/pros-and-cons-of-a-desk-cycle-2016-10?r=UK&IR=T

Protein. (2018, November 14). Retrieved from https://www.hsph.harvard.edu/nutritionsource/what-should-you-eat/protein/

Punching Bag Workout Benefits: 13 Reasons to Do Heavy Bag Training. (2018, March 20). Retrieved from https://fitbodybuzz.com/punching-bag-workout-benefits/

Quadriceps femoris muscle. (2018, November 27). Retrieved from https://en.wikipedia.org/wiki/Quadriceps_femoris_muscle

Raw vs Cooked Vegetables: The Healthiest Ways to Eat Your Veggies. (2018, September 06). Retrieved from https://foodrevolution.org/blog/food-and-health/raw-vs-cooked-vegetables/

Retrieved from https://www.google.com/search?q=how long does the average diet last&oq=how long does the average diet last&aqs=chrome..69i57.7376j0j7&sourceid=chrome&ie=UTF-8

Rettner, R. (2016, July 12). Lifting Weights? No Need to Go Heavy. Retrieved from https://www.livescience.com/55381-light-heavy-weights-muscle-strengthening.html

Ritterbeck, M. (2016, July 15). How to Do the Perfect Lunge. Retrieved from https://greatist.com/move/lunge-how-to-do-a-perfect-forward-lunge

Robinson, K. M. (n.d.). P90X: What to Expect from this DVD Workout. Retrieved from https://www.webmd.com/fitness-exercise/a-z/p90x-workout

Rogers, P. (n.d.). How Can You Exercise and Stretch the Hamstring Muscles? Retrieved from https://www.verywellfit.com/hamstring-muscle-anatomy-and-stretches-3498372

S, J., Allan, Backlin, B., Tomás, Holman, P., Tabitha, . . . CTS. (2018, September 17). Do Altitude Training Masks Work for Endurance Athletes? Retrieved from https://trainright.com/do-altitude-training-masks-work-for-endurance-athletes/

Saturated Fat. (n.d.). Retrieved from http://www.heart.org/en/healthy-living/healthy-eating/eat-smart/fats/saturated-fats

Saunas: Weight Loss Miracle? (n.d.). Retrieved from https://www.healthline.com/health/sauna-weight-loss-miracle#heart-health

Semeco, A. (2017). The Top 10 Benefits of Regular Exercise. [online] Healthline. Available at: https://www.healthline.com/nutrition/10-benefits-of-exercise [Accessed 25 Sep. 2018].

Shmerling, R. H. (2016, September 27). The truth behind standing desks. Retrieved from https://www.health.harvard.edu/blog/the-truth-behind-standing-desks-2016092310264

Shmerling, R. H. (2017, September 25). The latest scoop on the health benefits of coffee. Retrieved from https://www.health.harvard.edu/blog/the-latest-scoop-on-the-health-benefits-of-coffee-2017092512429

Simple Steps to Preventing Diabetes. (2016, July 25). Retrieved from https://www.hsph.harvard.edu/nutritionsource/disease-prevention/diabetes-prevention/preventing-diabetes-full-story/

Skarnulis, L. (n.d.). Jumping Rope Exercise Benefits: Burning Calories, Weight Loss. Retrieved from https://www.webmd.com/fitness-exercise/features/skipping-rope-doesnt-skip-workout#1

Soft Drinks and Disease. (2016, March 17). Retrieved from https://www.hsph.harvard.edu/nutritionsource/healthy-drinks/soft-drinks-and-disease/

Szalay, J. (2015, August 27). What Is Fiber? Retrieved from https://www.livescience.com/51998-dietary-fiber.html

Team, G. (2016, June 06). The 10-Minute Core-Blasting Pilates Workout. Retrieved from https://greatist.com/fitness/10-minute-pilates-workout

Tello, M. (2017, May 24). Run for your (long) life. Retrieved from https://www.health.harvard.edu/blog/run-long-life-2017052411722

The Average American Drinks How Much Soda per Year? (n.d.). Retrieved from http://www.madsenmed.com/blog/2017/7/5/-the-average-american-drinks-how-much-soda-per-year

The Impact of Obesity on Your Body and Health | ASMBS. (n.d.). Retrieved from https://asmbs.org/patients/impact-of-obesity

The Skinny on Fats. (n.d.). Retrieved from http://www.heart.org/en/health-topics/cholesterol/prevention-and-treatment-of-high-cholesterol-hyperlipidemia/the-skinny-on-fats

The Truth About Pre-Workout Supplements, Do They Really Work? (2018, March 04). Retrieved from https://www.foodforfitness.co.uk/pre-workout-supplements/

The Truth About Zero-Calorie Food. (2009, April 03). Retrieved from https://www.everydayhealth.com/weight/zero-calorie-food-myths.aspx

Tips for increasing physical activity. (2015, June 10). Retrieved from https://www.choosemyplate.gov/physical-activity-tips

Trans fat: Double trouble for your heart. (2017, March 01). Retrieved from https://www.mayoclinic.org/diseases-conditions/high-blood-cholesterol/in-depth/trans-fat/art-20046114

Trapezius Muscle. (n.d.). Retrieved from http://www.innerbody.com/image_musfov/musc28-new.html

Triglyceride. (2018, October 19). Retrieved from https://en.wikipedia.org/wiki/Triglyceride

Type 2 Diabetes: Symptoms, Causes, Diagnosis, and Prevention. (n.d.). Retrieved from https://www.webmd.com/diabetes/type-2-diabetes#1

Types of Fat. (2018, July 24). Retrieved from https://www.hsph.harvard.edu/nutritionsource/what-should-you-eat/fats-and-cholesterol/types-of-fat/

Ucl. (2018, November 15). How long does it take to form a habit? Retrieved from https://www.ucl.ac.uk/news/news-articles/0908/09080401

Veganism. (2018, December 21). Retrieved from https://en.wikipedia.org/wiki/Veganism

Villines, Z. (n.d.). CoolSculpting: Does it work and is it safe? Retrieved from https://www.medicalnewstoday.com/articles/322060.php

Vitamins. (2014, February 12). Retrieved from https://www.hsph.harvard.edu/nutritionsource/what-should-you-eat/vitamins/

Weight loss stalled? Move past the plateau. (2018, February 06). Retrieved from https://www.mayoclinic.org/healthy-lifestyle/weight-loss/in-depth/weight-loss-plateau/art-20044615

What does "Non GMO" mean? (2017, August 07). Retrieved from http://greenerchoices.org/2017/03/07/non-gmo-mean/

What exactly is a calorie? | Discover Good Nutrition. (2016, December 29). Retrieved from https://discovergoodnutrition.com/2015/06/what-is-a-calorie/

Zelman, K. M. (n.d.). Why Drink More Water? See 6 Health Benefits of Water. Retrieved from https://www.webmd.com/diet/features/6-reasons-to-drink-water#1